WHY
HUMAN RIGHTS
IN CHILDBIRTH
MATTER

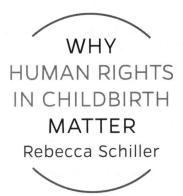

WHY
HUMAN RIGHTS
IN CHILDBIRTH
MATTER
Rebecca Schiller

Why Human Rights in Childbirth Matter (Pinter & Martin Why It Matters 9)

First published by Pinter & Martin Ltd 2016

© 2016 Rebecca Schiller

Rebecca Schiller has asserted her moral right to be identified as the author of this work in accordance with the Copyright, Designs and Patents Act of 1988.

All rights reserved

ISBN 978-1-78066-580-1

Also available as ebook

Pinter & Martin Why It Matters ISSN 2056-8657
Series editor: Susan Last
Index: Helen Bilton
Design: Rebecca Longworth
Cover Design: Blok Graphic, London
Cover illustration: Donna Smith
Proofreader: Debbie Kennett

British Library Cataloguing-in-Publication Data

A catalogue record for this book is available from the British Library.

This book is sold subject to the condition that it shall not, by way of trade and otherwise, be lent, resold, hired out, or otherwise circulated without the publisher's prior consent in any form or binding or cover other than that in which it is published and without a similar condition being imposed on the subsequent purchaser.

Set in Minion

Printed and bound in the UK by Ashford Colour Press Ltd, Gosport, Hampshire

This book has been printed on paper that is sourced and harvested from sustainable forests and is FSC accredited.

Pinter & Martin Ltd
6 Effra Parade
London SW2 1PS
pinterandmartin.com

Contents

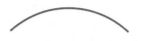

Author's Note

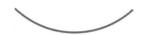

In a short book on a huge topic there are inevitable generalisations that don't reflect the uniqueness of each experience across the spectrum of childbirth. For this I apologise in advance.

Throughout I will use a mixture of ways to refer to those who go through pregnancy and birth, acknowledging that not all people with uteruses identify with the term woman. I will also use the term 'woman' but want to acknowledge that reproductive rights and the experiences around them are, of course, pertinent for transgender and gender non-conforming people who may not identify with that term. I use it with awareness that it cannot contain the identities of a number of people to whom all or parts of it may apply.

Partners (fathers in particular), and the role of family more broadly, are again sidelined here. This is partly for reasons of space, but also because I believe it is important to tackle these issues first from the perspective of the key protagonist in the room – who should always be the person giving birth.

Some of the stories, examples and discussions in this book may be triggering for those with previous birth trauma, a history of sexual abuse or those who are living with the ongoing impact of a range of traumas.

I've chosen to look at issues around the world, believing that human rights in childbirth, and broader reproductive rights, are viewed more clearly with knowledge across, and access to, more than one part of the spectrum. Shining a spotlight on issues in other countries could have a positive impact on women closer to home. Insisting on local women being treated with dignity and respect should also ripple out to others far away. Despite that, the specific legal framework discussed in this book is often based around English law, though the underlying principles and issues are pertinent to global readers. Signposts to more global information are to be found in the 'Resources and Further Reading' section at the end of the book.

Finally, I want to acknowledge that many of us, including myself, have had resoundingly positive experiences of pregnancy, birth and new parenthood. There are numerous obstetricians, midwives, academics, campaigners, doulas, lawyers, journalists and more working to guard and expand these positive realities across the world. It is important to bring the many challenges and inequalities to light, but I firmly believe that, in almost every case, problems are systemic and cultural and not the fault of individual practitioners.

I thank all those working hard to tip the scales for their work, which often goes without recognition. This book is dedicated to them, the women who have shared these most intimate of moments with me, and my husband and children for opening my eyes to another world.

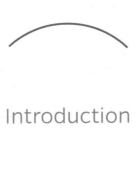

Introduction

I am sitting at my desk wondering how I came to be a human rights in childbirth activist. There are tiny, crisp moments in my life that stand out. I roll them around my mind like grains of salt across a palm. Minutes of time that I could have forgotten, but instead have left their residue across my life. Tangy and sharp-edged. It was inevitable that I'd choose this work eventually.

It was me sitting next to that girl at school. The one being picked on because she was different. Hating unfairness to the point of tears. I discovered what rage felt like when a teenage classmate told me that women who had abortions were evil and would go to hell. The idea that something arbitrary could be used to stop a vulnerable group exercising a basic right, or judge them harshly if they did, set something up in my brain. A little alarm that then went off when I saw the pattern repeated.

Travelling in Bosnia with a university friend I became interested in human rights in war. I held in my hands the names of 8,000 men and boys massacred at Srebrenica in 1995 – a dossier painstakingly compiled by one of their mothers. It was all that was left of her son and his fellow victims. In presenting each of the names and asking us to read them she reminded us of the lost individual. She took us behind the horror of the number '8,000' to see that there were human beings here who should have been entitled to more. Exposing their humanity to show us why the lives of individuals matter.

Then, much later, in my work as a doula, I saw incredible strength, superb care, enduring compassion, love, support and professional excellence. The very best of life squared up to some of the worst. My injustice alarm began to ring and it is yet to stop. I found out that words like 'woman-centred' were thrown around easily, but were often weighted down with a heavy burden of women being put firmly in their place.

In birth rooms I witnessed things that I could barely believe could happen in contemporary England. The tendrils of a patriarchy I'd never realised had much to do with me were so firmly entangled in maternity care. I'd been lucky enough never to personally experience how fragile the illusion of women playing a full and equal part in society was. But here, in a context where I wasn't looking for it, was the evidence.

The 'Am I allowed?' question came out of pregnant women's mouths with alarming regularity. The answer from the system was often 'no'. The power balance in birth, the negative political and moral discourse around women's agency in reproduction, the repeated judgements, pressures and constraints: I didn't have to do more than creep in to a couple of labour wards to see them all laid bare.

There is one birthing woman I will never forget. I watched her shout 'no' repeatedly while fingers, then instruments, were repeatedly inserted into her vagina. There was no ambiguity about her wishes and no attempt to defer to them.

She did not give consent, but they carried on regardless. As if she was inanimate.

I held her hand and soothed her, feeling complicit. Not knowing how to stop what was clearly an abusive crime presented as a matter of routine. Something that 'good girls' should endure for the sake of their babies. I realised that these abuses were repeated to a greater and lesser degree every day and that we weren't allowed to complain about it. If we did, we would be sucked in to a distracting vortex of ideological birth talk. Women against women, arguing about birth pools vs epidurals and whether caesareans or free births were a safer or a more 'empowered' way of giving birth. Constantly steered away from the real issues around women's autonomy in birth.

So when I met Elizabeth Prochaska, an inspiring human rights barrister with an interest in maternity care, everything began to drop neatly into place. Elizabeth had been doing some pro bono (volunteer) work giving legal advice to midwives. She rang me to tell me that she had just succeeded in ensuring that a local NHS Trust provided independent midwives to women while the NHS homebirth service was suspended. I had a client deeply affected by the service suspension and Elizabeth's work meant that, instead of having to overcome a significant fear of hospital, Jennymay birthed at home with midwives she had time to get to know and who returned to care for her postnatally. There was real power in what Elizabeth was doing.

At the amazing first Human Rights in Childbirth conference at The Hague in 2012 Elizabeth told me she was thinking of starting a charity to house her pro bono maternity-focused work. A place where the human rights principles and framework could be used to improve maternity care. We started Birthrights in January 2013 with a board of lawyers, midwives, doctors and service users to drive change forwards.

And since 2015 I have been its chief executive.

Over the past three years my outlook on and focus within the birth world has changed. I've moved away from some of what drew me in and in some instances entirely changed my opinion. I make no apology for that, but the process of doing so has been difficult and at times I've wondered how I could reconcile the different areas of my work.

In some ways this book is a selfish attempt to stitch my different interests and perspectives together. To think about why rights in childbirth are violated. To place these rights in their broader context as part of the feminist project and wider reproductive rights movement. To show why this matters and to understand how the human rights framework might make the kind of progress in childbirth that has proved too much for other approaches. To tease out the contradictions, find the sticky corners where we often get trapped and to try to find a message we can agree on so that, despite our contrasting experiences and our different personal and political preferences, we can move forward together.

I've divided the book into two sections. The first explores these issues and draws conclusions. This is the section I hope you'll find thought-provoking and even challenging at times. You'll notice I spend some time thinking about the place of childbirth in our world today before moving on to talk about human rights more explicitly. I think this scene-setting is important and though the phrase 'human rights' is only lightly sprinkled across the first two chapters, the focus on the tension between the individual, the rest of the world, the state and its systems is inherent to these chapters just as it is to the human rights movement.

The second section is more practical: your pocket guide to what women's rights in birth really are. Covering the basics and then looking at specific areas of tension, it will help you understand and use the human rights legal framework to ensure that your own rights in pregnancy and birth are protected. If you are a midwife, doctor or birth worker I hope it will help you to reinforce what the maternity system should provide, complement and make more powerful the work you do providing safe, quality, respectful care to the women you meet, while helping you to understand your obligations.

This second section (and indeed the entire book) owes a great debt to the legal expertise of Elizabeth Prochaska and a number of Birthrights volunteers, who have produced a range of clear, concise factsheets on human rights in childbirth that are available at birthrights.org.uk. I thank her and them for what they do, which is always useful and makes things happen.

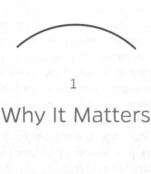

1
Why It Matters

On 6 October 2013 I caught my second baby as he slid out of me. There he was, my newborn son. The misshapen head that often characterises vaginal birth. The still-separate plates of his soft skull moulded to the shape of my birth canal. There was no point being made, no ethos being followed, no agenda. Just life happening. A huge experience in my life. The first in his.

It was very quiet in the half-second until he cried. Just my husband and me, somewhat shellshocked, alone in the house. Then he opened his mouth and eyes looking for my face. My personal kaleidoscope had turned and all that was in view was the two of us.

For a birth in the UK mine is unusual. No one told me what to do or what not to do. Like 48 million women around the world each year, according to Save the Children,[1] I had given birth without a skilled attendant. Unlike the majority of them, I had an independent midwife racing through the countryside towards me. In contrast to two million women each year across the world I was not completely alone.

Twenty minutes before I gave birth I turned to my husband and said: 'It's going to be just you and me.' Out of nowhere, minutes after labour had started, my body was efficiently spitting out the baby it had kept safe until its 'due date'. I felt a little afraid as the world shifted inside me at an incredible pace. I knew the baby was fine, but I wanted my midwife and doula by my side to look me in the eyes and tell me I could do this impossible task. I didn't plan it this way.

He came twisting and turning through my pelvis into the world. Everyday, staggering, amazing and awful all together. This was something that happened to me and him. In ways he is unaware of, his birth may shape parts of his life. In more obvious ways, it will be marked on my body and woven into my personal narrative.

As a mirror to society, childbirth, the attitudes to it, practices around it and experiences of women going through it, reflect the progress that has been made in advancing women's rights. This reflection also shows us that there's still a long road ahead. But right then I wasn't looking in the mirror. I was gently holding a little purple body against my skin and stroking his damp face. A birth is as private as you can get. My baby's birth. My birth. Ours. His. Mine.

Like so many of us, I became interested in human rights quite simply because injustice makes me angry and I care about people. Later, I had my first baby and I thought I had found a different vocation: supporting women and their families through pregnancy and birth. It didn't take long to realise that my two career pathways were linked in a number of ways.

Childbirth and human rights have taken time to find each other, despite the fact that our humanity, and the rights conferred on us by it, is ignited in the moment our mothers push us out of their bodies. It is hard to be confident about freedom and safety when we are born in a context of disrespect, abuse or neglect.

However, the rights of individuals in childbirth are not simply reflective of broader attitudes. They are fundamental to protecting our freedoms, and both birth and feminist campaigners are beginning to see how powerful getting it right or wrong in birth can be. Researching this book, along with my wider work supporting women and campaigning, has convinced me that we cannot progress a women's rights agenda without tackling the particular rights within this unique experience. After all, birth can only happen to someone with female reproductive organs, and 84 per cent of women get pregnant and give birth at some point in their lives. Lynn Paltrow, of the US organisation National Advocates for Pregnant Women (NAPW), believes that 'advocating for pregnant women is advocating for all women and their human rights'. After all, she continues, 'It is women's capacity for pregnancy that is used as the excuse for differential treatment.' Whether or not pregnancy and birth are on our individual radar, the position of women in society – often playing a different and lesser role in political, social and economic arenas – stems from this capacity.

Our ability to become pregnant is the root excuse for treating women as second-class citizens. The punishments, control, surveillance and barriers to full and equal participation in society are imposed disproportionately, says Paltrow, on those who are vulnerable for economic, racial or other reasons. As maternal and neonatal mortality statistics and the experiences of women in the forthcoming chapters show, some are more prone to discrimination than others. They face more physical and emotional dangers within the pregnancy and child-bearing process, which are reflective of, intertwined with and in some ways propel the difficulties they face in their other interactions with society.

Getting it right in the birth context could provide a strong platform from which to assert how vital it is that all women are treated as humans at all times, with the rights this should afford them. By contrast, childbirth also provides the perfect opportunity to undermine those rights. Looking across the developed and developing world it is clear that the broad spectrum of women's freedoms is undermined daily in birth. If we don't value their experiences in an act that is particular to them, we make it an easy access point for those who seek to disrupt feminist progress.

Assumptions that would be challenged in other contexts seem to persist in childbirth. The spectre of foetal rights is an ill-conceived yet easily wielded tool to distract from punitive measures that target vulnerable pregnant women strategically to undermine women's rights more broadly. An anti-woman culture promotes an antagonistic discourse around birth and motherhood. It turns our eyes from serious back-pedalling on basic reproductive freedoms, and exploits the emotive experience of identity and mothering to our disadvantage.

There is much to be concerned about and I am not being hyperbolic when I say that what is happening in the US to women's reproductive rights, often via the back door of undefended birth rights, is terrifying. There is also much cause for hope, with grassroots action rising up to meet top-down recognition of these issues with some real effect.

This book is about birth, but beyond that it is simply about the human rights of women. Feminism has touched on birth across its history but, as Human Rights in Childbirth founder Hermine Hayes-Klein notes, it is only now that progress has been made in other areas that the current wave of feminists is able and beginning to engage with it fully. To succeed, we must all see human rights in childbirth as fundamental to protecting the entire spectrum of reproductive freedoms.

I will argue that we all need to take note of childbirth; whatever our gender, whatever our plans for children, whatever our past experience. I will talk about it as an essentially personal event and will tell some of those individual stories from around the world. In highlighting the individual nature of the experience, I hope to show why it is childbirth's very individuality, and the protection of that, which should prompt us to engage with it collectively, and how the human rights framework can be used to navigate the tension between personal and societal needs.

At the heart of this is a question about the statement that is frequently the mantra of contemporary, developed world birth: is all that matters a healthy baby? Say it often enough and perhaps it becomes true. Pregnant people say it when explaining their birth choices. Some doctors and midwives lightly tack it on to coercive discussions. Friends and family say it, often in consolation, after a difficult birth. In the moments after my son's birth, it was all that mattered to me.

Of course, it is true in many moments for many women. There's little research on the matter, but Mary Nolan, professor of perinatal education, believes that most women who decide to continue with their pregnancies are driven to keep their babies safe. Be it biological programming or cultural conditioning, in most circumstances women are determined to see their babies happily into the outside world. A healthy baby may be all that matters to them in certain moments.

Yet when I, in my immediate post-birth, mammal-like state, had zoomed in entirely on my new son, it was in an important context. When I say 'my healthy baby was all that matters', I am leaving out much, expecting it to be taken as read. That I am incredibly privileged in so many ways. That I had consented to the sex that conceived the baby. That I had access to contraception if I had wanted it. That I decided I wanted to continue with the pregnancy and had access to free, safe abortion if I hadn't. That I lived in a country that offered me free, expert maternity care should I want it. That I could, just about, afford to pay an independent midwife when I realised the system might not work for me. That I would retain autonomy to make the decisions that I felt were best for me, my baby and my family. That no one would intentionally hurt me while I was in labour, or threaten me, or bully me, or take me to court and strap me against my will to an operating table and cut me open if I declined a suggested course of action. That after my baby was born I would be cared for, offered support, have access to life-saving drugs in case of haemorrhage. That I would matter.

The myth that 'a healthy baby is all that matters' needs to be unpicked. It cannot be left as read because, where the assumptions go unchallenged, a frightening and reductive world begins to appear. A world in which so many individuals cannot expect all the things I have listed above, and where backwards steps in women's rights to freedom and justice are being made, often couched in the flawed logic of protecting the unborn but failing by their very nature to do so.

I want to say that a healthy baby is not all that matters and that, resoundingly, *it all matters*. Human rights in childbirth matter. This is the story of women, of why they matter too, and the things that happen when they are pushed to the bottom of a hierarchy in birth.

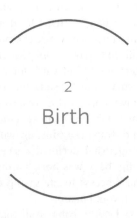

2
Birth

Momentous and ordinary

Birth happens so frequently that it should be dull, yet it retains its miraculous status. Like death, it is one of the core human experiences and one that unites us with the other 5,416 species of mammals. Like them, the birth of our infants is governed by an interplay of hormones. Our physiologies work best when we feel safe and unobserved. And, again like other mammals, the realities of life mean that our infants are frequently born in less than ideal circumstances, our bodies coping as best they can.

One of the truisms applied to birth is its simultaneously momentous and routine nature. Aside from our own births, most of us will be present at the birth of another during our lives. Some 1,900 babies are born in the UK each day. Around 10,800 come into the world daily in the US and 353,000 globally. It is not just part of life, it *is* life. Day in, day out, extraordinary and ordinary stories that will be remembered for a lifetime have their very first telling.

In developed countries childbirth now happens on average less than twice in our lifetimes. Within the lives of individuals, the consequences of birth are huge and the impact of the event itself profound. It is remarkable because on the micro level it is a life-altering rarity.

Birth's status as a crucial event may be influenced partly by its historical position. Harriet Blodgett's look at centuries of female diarists points to birth as a 'time of excitement, competition and deep fear'. It was previously analogous to the battlefield experience for men, bringing with it the 'likelihood of suffering, not to mention the possibility of death' that was seen as fundamental in building character.[2] Our ancestors' relationship with childbirth was based heavily on the reality of dying during it. Worryingly, today in the developing world some countries' maternal mortality rates warrant similar levels of fear.

In the UK, where childbirth now brings with it a very tiny risk of death (0.0086 per cent of women) the intense focus on and fear of birth can't be explained in the same way. Academic Alison Phipps thinks that there is a particular intensity around how birth and new motherhood are presented right now, and that this is the result of a number of different forces. She explains that 'we've lost that important notion of the "good enough" mother and we're all striving to be the perfect mother'. She points to the individualisation of responsibility that comes as a package with our neoliberal healthcare system, noting the pressure we're under 'to produce the best children that we possibly can while being as little of a drain on the health service'. Pregnancy and birth as the gateway to perfect motherhood, dragging behind them the historical shadow of death, can understandably weigh heavily on the mind, the policymaker and the media.

Becoming a mother can feel all-consuming, and society

often encourages us to believe that this new part of our identity has eclipsed our old self entirely. Phipps thinks this is tied to a pervasive anti-feminist drive that seeks to reinforce traditional gender roles by putting particular emphasis on motherhood. 'There's a feeling', she has observed, 'that if you do it wrong at any point all hell will break loose.' Perhaps this had trickled down to the health visitors I saw after my first baby was born, who almost religiously avoided using my name and referred to me only as 'Mum'. It's a trend that more than one commentator has remarked on. American columnist and author Heather Havrilsky has written about her loss of individual identity after becoming a mother, noting the number of people now addressing her as 'Mom'. She feels that 'motherhood is no longer viewed as simply a relationship with your children' and that it has been 'elevated – or perhaps demoted – to the realm of lifestyle, an all-encompassing identity with demands and expectations that eclipse everything else in a woman's life'.[3]

Childbirth, and the pregnancy that precedes it, is positioned as a passageway to a brand-new life. Not just for babies, but for those who grow them. Contemporary developed world systems, while largely achieving a very low risk of death, add new layers of import and place the burden of responsibility on the mother to get it right or else. A daunting task when, unlike our ancestors, many of us experience birth for the first time only when we are actually doing it ourselves.

A complex record of society

Elizabeth L'Estrange's analysis of 14th- and 15th-century birthing chamber charms, amulets and incantations[4] locates birth as a spiritual, religious and mysterious experience as well as an event in the lives of our ancestors. In the 21st-century UK it could be argued that breathing techniques, hypnobirthing scripts and a range of obstetric and midwifery rituals fulfil similar roles.

Yet birth's mysterious nature is perhaps most obviously highlighted by scientists' failure to fully unravel how it actually works. The question of what triggers labour is still contested. A long-held belief that babies are born just before their head circumferences grow too large to fit through the pelvis is going out of fashion. Professor Shaun Brennecke points to a protein prompt that switches on contractions,[5] while Dr Carole Mendelson suggests that a chemical signal is given to the mother once the unborn's lungs are sufficiently mature.[6] A new theory from the University of Rhode Island speculates that babies are born when their mother's metabolic rate can no longer support their growth.[7] In short, no one knows.

The implications of the complex series of hormonal processes that govern birth and bonding are also still being understood. Dr Kerstin Uvnäs Moberg's research into the role of oxytocin (one of the most fundamental hormones that governs birth, breastfeeding and human bonding) provides an interesting theory that our hormone set-up at birth could impact on our capacity to form relationships for the rest of our lives.[8] Obstetrician Michel Odent takes this a step further, hypothesising that contemporary birth practices cause us to use our hormonal systems less, resulting in a diminishing effectiveness of our physiology generation by generation. Odent feels that epigenetic consequences may lead to a future where we are simply unable to give birth without intervention.[9] Meanwhile, in the fields of microbiology and immunology, much-contested ideas are emerging that describe a link between long-term health (and in particular the huge rise in non-communicable diseases) and bacterial seeding that happens during and immediately after birth.[10]

We know far more than we did 100 years ago, but more still is beyond us and even more is subject to argument and confusion. Childbirth still has its mysteries and they are slow to make themselves known. For individuals making decisions about their own pregnancies and births, the stakes are high, the impact is significant and the information is often oppositional. For women, at the mercy of a culture that places huge responsibility yet often a lack of respect on the mother figure, birth can become loaded with extra significance, especially when theories and grade A evidence are presented as if they are one and the same.

Author and radical doula Elisa Albert notes, 'it's become fashionable to obscure the question of how we give birth as a matter of personal preference rather than a systemic problem with real public-health consequences.'[11] Magnifying this is a media whose interest in birth is matched only by its positioning of the event as entirely dichotomised in a way that's usually unfriendly to the women it represents. Some are 'too posh to push'. Others are risk-taking homebirth hippies. Perhaps this is in part a natural by-product of the media focus (after all, antagonism makes a better story). But it's far more complex than that. Antagonism is inherent in stories of birth because motherhood means so much to us. It feels personal when someone challenges our way of doing things, or questions our beliefs. Moreover, the broader cultural implications of a still-patriarchal society put women in competition with each other, as Phipps adds, 'almost as a way to distract us from the broader inequalities we live with in relation to men'.

The effects of these interlocking forces that highlight pregnancy and birth within our culture and identities are hard to map, but in British women giving birth today levels of fear appear to be on the rise. In 2003 midwifery professor Josephine Green and colleagues compared women's experiences of childbirth from 1987 to 2000. The research demonstrated that 10–12 per cent more mothers described themselves as frightened in 2000 than only 13 years earlier. For first-time mothers there was a depressing 12 per cent rise in feeling 'overwhelmed' and more women felt 'out of control', 'challenged', 'helpless', 'detached' and 'powerless'. Many fewer felt 'excited' or 'confident', and the greatest shift was shown when women were asked if they felt 'involved' in their experience of childbirth, with the figure dropping from 42 per cent in 1987 to 28 per cent in 2000.[12]

The way we as individuals and societies approach birth is all at once a complex record of a precise point in time, our unique and collective histories, our beliefs, practices and social mores, among many other things. While it may be of concern that so much has moved in a negative direction in a short space of time, it is normal that attitudes and experiences change. I agree with anthropologist Sheila Kitzinger when she commented that 'choices about birth are never as simple as selecting a can of beans from a supermarket shelf'. She pointed to the powerful emotions involved, explaining: 'It is understandable that this should be so because birth is not just a matter of pushing a baby out of your body, a demonstration of bio-mechanics, but concerns fundamental human values.'[13]

Public property

While fear grows among women, and scrutiny of mothers increases, maternity care has become a public health priority across the developed and developing world. In 1902, the UK passed the Midwives Act, which was probably the first serious attempt to address maternity issues in a structured, public way. Though largely set up to regulate midwifery in response to concerns for infant welfare, the act represents a step towards bringing childbirth inside a system.

Today, a myriad of government, non-governmental, medical, midwifery, campaigner, peer, research and other local, national and international organisations have something to say about how birth should be. While there are broad trends (including an aim to reduce caesarean rates and increase vaginal birth and breastfeeding), the ambitions of these groups are often oppositional. The process of and reaction to the recent National Maternity Review in England serves as a classic example of the tangled complexities involved in trying to improve birth.

In this context the individual decisions I made during my pregnancy are not as individual as I would have them. I have been influenced by the media, my peers and my family, and I translated this into something that feels unique to me. Crucially, my decisions are now made within a broader context of what is recommended by official bodies and where they place their emphasis and funds. There may be a conflict between what I want and what society says is best.

Admitting that our approaches to life are not as individual as we would like to believe is not the same as agreeing that we are happy to relinquish personal control altogether. However, childbirth and the experiences around it are increasingly loaded with political significance, subject to moral scrutiny and part of a bigger picture. Individuals find themselves by accident inside a statistic, outside a guideline, falling in with a public health initiative and identifying with a constructed tribe. A tribe whose values they often feel they must accept completely in order to give them a map with which to navigate the challenging terrain that this new life-stage brings.

So while I stand by my assertion that birth is essentially a personal story, the wider interest and implications cannot be ignored. Birth is interesting, important. It is an 'issue'; sometimes it's a cause, at other times a problem, a battle, a case for investment. The public lens wants to view childbirth and rightly so. It needs to report on it, improve it, save money and lives, and within that the essential privacy of individual decisions and journeys becomes lost. There is a tension between the personal experience of birth and birth as public property. Stretched uncomfortably between these poles are women across the world. Within that discomfort and the reactions to it, is much that helps us understand the world around us and the inherent difficulties women face when interacting with it. I will go on to argue that a human rights approach can be a crucial tool in managing this tension.

Looking at how a society approaches childbirth, how it constructs a system around it, the rituals, the rites and the way it treats the key protagonist – the birthing woman – is akin to taking the temperature of that society. Nothing says more about the communities we live in than how they treat their most vulnerable at this extraordinary time. Outside of our own birth stories and lives, birth as a topic is rich and deep.

Ideas about childbirth have always been fluid, but never has birth changed as rapidly and comprehensively as in the developed world over the past 150 years. The industrialisation of childbirth happened much later than other forms of industrialisation. In the UK, much took place after the advent of the NHS, with roots trailing back past the beginning of the 20th century. From then, childbirth moved at a lightning pace from being a primarily home-based, locally centred, social experience to one almost exclusively centralised in large-scale obstetric units, bringing tangible benefits but also interrelated drawbacks.

Professor Mavis Kirkham, an academic with over 40 years' practical midwifery experience, believes that childbirth in the UK today has not yet moved into its post-industrial phase, explaining that 'women and workers still experience it as a conveyor belt, though it is moving rather faster than it used to'. She describes a system that is 'becoming more rigid because the working culture is full of blame and fear' and that the management of maternity services is obsessive about 'its need to control'.

A more recent focus on returning midwifery, birth and other related services to the community (most prominently in the 2016 National Review of Maternity Services in England)[14] has not yet prompted much tangible change and has often been met with suspicion by campaign groups, healthcare professionals, media and women. Their caution is perhaps unsurprising, given the entirely opposite messaging of the past 100 years and the current structure of the maternity services.

The systemising of maternity care has been dealt with differently in every country, subject to the cultural context and infrastructure. In the USA today only 7.9 per cent of births are attended by midwives, with over 90 per cent of women having obstetric-led care including support from an obstetric nurse. In the UK, by contrast, the majority of women have care from a midwife and significant midwifery involvement in their births. Swedish mothers are routinely offered only one ultrasound during their pregnancies, whereas in France they are normally given three and 20 per cent have more than six.[15] In the Netherlands, 20 per cent[16] of women give birth at home. In Australia that figure is 0.9 per cent.[17] In the UK the episiotomy (a cut made in a woman's perineum) rate is 19.4 per cent.[18] In Italy, despite evidence discouraging its routine use, the rate is 43.6 per cent,[19] for reasons that Italian consultant obstetrician Elena Cesari describes as 'traditional and cultural'. In Cyprus a staggering 75 per cent of women have an episiotomy, of which the vast majority must be entirely unnecessary.[20] A March 2016 report by the Royal College of Obstetricians and Gynaecologists highlighted some significant variations within England too – notably a 15 per cent difference in episiotomy rates across the country.[21]

These statistics alone highlight the impact of non-evidence-based forces on maternity systems, practices and ultimately women's bodies. A detailed examination of global differences would more than fill this book.

For me, though, pregnancy and birth, despite its broader context, is principally still something that happens or doesn't happen to an individual woman. A personal decision to have children or to keep an accidental pregnancy. An easy journey or one that requires fertility assistance. Planning not to have children is, of course, just as valid a choice, and some women may be desperate for children but find it impossible to conceive. More than ever before there are a range of pathways that lead one in five women to a life without children and the rest to childbirth.

For the four-fifths of women who experience it, giving birth in the developed world today has much to recommend it. The overwhelming majority of women have access to antenatal care from experts able to offer intervention to keep the baby and mother safe. In the UK, this care is provided free to almost all and, when the time arrives, women are able (at least theoretically) to choose where to give birth and will be supported by knowledgeable clinicians keen to ensure a safe outcome.

Medical intervention is saving lives on a daily basis. Babies born as early as 24 weeks are sometimes able to live. Mothers with complex heart problems or serious conditions such as pre-eclampsia, which a hundred years ago would have meant an almost certain death, can now be treated. Post-birth haemorrhages that would have proved fatal are controlled with synthetic hormones. Caregivers are aware of the importance of hand-washing and of using sterile equipment. Where in the developing world babies might die from infection in the umbilical cord stump, access to sterile equipment and antibiotics ensures the same doesn't happen here.

So why – despite the fact that the 2011 Birthplace in England study[22] showed that giving birth in the UK is incredibly safe for mother and baby – is fear on the rise?

A healthy baby

They wheeled me along, through double doors, just like you imagine. Everyone was happy though and I got happy too. I was no longer oppressed. I was liberating myself from the tyranny of the body. And then, there I was, in the room. I couldn't believe how much like an operating room it felt. Cold, bright lights, antiseptic, people scurrying around and chatting with each other. It was like being present at my own death. It was horrific but wonderful, too. I felt at peace in a way, like things were being taken care of, finally. This I could endure. Dustin sat on a stool near my head and held my hand, tangled in IVs. We cried; I shook. His surgical mask was wet with tears and snot. Our baby. His baby. I felt that the first time, then.

'OK,' she said, tapping me, 'they're going to start pushing him out! It's going to feel really weird, OK? But that's normal.' She held my right hand, Dustin my left. They started to tug. The force of it had my half-dead body swaying like a canoe. My eyes, I'm sure, got huge. I stared straight ahead as if to focus on the task at hand. Not scream, to not use whatever strength I had left to fling myself off the operating table. The task was to endure the most bizarre experience of my life, the feeling, painless, of someone yanking all of your organs out. I am a vessel, only. I am something to be pillaged. I am a cabinet, a pantry door. I am lying naked on a table in a

cold room under bright lights, my arms splayed out to form a T, and a team of people are gathered around my body, peering in.

And then I heard a cry.

What I felt then, above all, was recognition. This isn't possible, it's an incorrect feeling if feelings can be described that way, but this was the part of my brain that lit up. His cry was like a familiar face in the crowd. I was lying on my back staring at the ceiling, shaking, with tears streaming down the sides of my cheeks. His cry, I was surprised to find, sounded like him. He sounded like his own person, distinct. Before then all baby cries sounded the same to me, but his cry was a voice. A self.

'So, they're basically putting you back together right now,' the anaesthesiologist said to me, matter-of-factly. I appreciated her honesty. The horror of it felt appropriate. I nodded, brave. All of it felt right, actually; to become a mother like this.[23]

I spend a lot of my time listening to stories of childbirth. In my work as a campaigner and doula, birth stories and witnessing birth are simply part of the job. In my social life, women tell me their birth stories often within minutes of being introduced once they realise I am interested.

Many of us have happy memories of giving birth to our children. Most, like writer Meaghan O'Connell above (who gave birth in March 2014 in New York), have complex tales; full of joy, fear, excitement and pain. Often, though, women seek me out because they are upset by what happened in the birth room. Very often they start their story with something like 'Of course I know all that really matters is that she's healthy, but...' The little tag tacked on to a narrative that is often very little about the baby and all about the woman, how she was treated and how she felt. By dismissing their own importance, prioritising their baby, confessing that they don't matter, they give themselves permission to talk about themselves. Perhaps this is natural, but I think it's also symptomatic of what academics like Dr Ellie Lee have called a rise in 'intensive motherhood'. It as though contemporary mothers have to acknowledge their slide down the hierarchy before they can be honest.

If in retrospect the baby is very understandably all that matters to its mother, is that something we should reinforce or, as a society and in our maternity services, should we be looking out for her as she looks out for her baby? The answer seems simple at first. Women grow babies. On one level it is impossible to say that 'a healthy baby is all that matters', because without a woman, at best a healthy woman, a baby would simply not exist. Yet by this logic women become important merely as containers, the vessel that Meaghan briefly describes herself to be. Something to be cared for because of its contents, but not because of its intrinsic value. That is something many of us find difficult to subscribe to; especially as, behind the faulty logic, there is often a far more telling and sometimes sinister story.

Lucy Jolin of the Birth Trauma Association feels that the phrase and sentiments behind it are 'often used as a way of minimising serious mental health issues and indirect victim-blaming', and that 'the ideal outcome is a mother and baby who are both healthy in both body and mind'. So what happens to women whose experiences of childbirth are in some way 'unhealthy' for them?

Popular opinion says that we soon forget the details of childbirth, but research shows that this is far from true. Sheila Kitzinger described how a woman in her 80s rang her 'Birth Crisis' helpline in tears to discuss her traumatic birth, which had taken place over 50 years earlier. Penny Simkin (founder of Doulas of North America) interviewed women who attended her childbirth classes over 20 years ago and found that their memories of childbirth were strong, accurate and sometimes 'strikingly vivid'[24] even two decades later.

Research from Japan[25] studied memories of births that had taken place five years earlier in detail, concluding that they were amazingly accurate. Childbirth persists in women's minds, often vividly, for a lifetime. More than that, though, its significance can affect their sense of self, their relationships with their children, their partners, their future ability to interact with healthcare services, their physical and emotional wellbeing and more. A 2013 Birthrights survey[26] of over 1,100 Mumsnet users found that those who characterised their baby's birth as a negative experience were far more likely to feel that it made them have negative thoughts about themselves and their babies.

Reports of post-traumatic stress disorder after birth range from 1.5 to 6 per cent, with a much higher number of women experiencing some symptoms of trauma. Cheryl Beck's 2004 study into this trauma reflects the findings of a number of others. Trauma isn't necessarily directly related to a particular kind of birth, but more to the way the birth is conducted. I agree with Jolin, who believes that an emergency caesarean section, if it is conducted in a way that enables the labouring mother to feel in control and respected, does not have to be traumatic. By contrast, a vaginal birth where she feels out of control and is not treated with respect may lead to trauma. And vice versa. Lack of control, insufficient pain relief, absence of respect and failure to pass on information are all major factors.

Childbirth's impact on women can be fundamental, though longitudinal research into the effects across women's lives is patchy at best. What is available shows that when a woman's childbirth experience is viewed through a negative lens it can have significant implications for her emotional wellbeing, aside from the physical challenges and changes that pregnancy and birth can bring. This is particularly compelling in light of the UK's Confidential Enquiry into Maternal Deaths,[27] which previously found the leading cause of maternal death to be suicide. Thankfully, in the latest enquiry the rate has dropped a little, but suicide is mentioned 85 times in the report and psychiatric causes of maternal death are still notable in number.

Positive effects of birth are also deeply felt by many women. In the studies and survey above, women who characterised childbirth in a positive way also felt good about themselves and their babies. How a woman feels during birth, and crucially how she is treated (including, but not limited to, whether she feels physically safe), is important for her wellbeing in the long term. Professor Kirkham believes that 'birth can transform our stories' and the qualitative and quantitative evidence is on her side. We need to be concerned that for so many women, their individual experience is one of fear and long-term upset. It is in looking at childbirth through the eyes of the individual that we see the fundamental human rights that can underpin a safe and positive experience of birth. And when they are absent or violated the threat to human dignity is all too real.

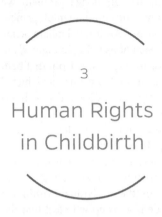

3

Human Rights in Childbirth

What are human rights?

In October 2014 the *Daily Express* front page proclaimed 'Human Rights Madness to End'. I was standing in a queue at the supermarket when I caught sight of it. There we all were with our trollies full of food, the vast majority going back to our adequate housing. Walking past the free schooling our children have access to and hoping not to fall and need the cushion of our health service, but knowing it was there if we did. The irony made me laugh and then crumple a little inside, as I do every time human rights are so misunderstood.

Next to the *Express* was the *Guardian*'s front page, with a very different headline, and next to that another and another. All of us in the supermarket free to say what we liked as long as it doesn't harm another, to choose which paper to buy and which politician to back. Dressing as we wanted, driving cars (even the women), expressing our sexual identities as we saw fit. Knowing we wouldn't be arbitrarily killed, or locked up without cause or trial. Human rights madness, eh?

Human rights has an image problem which belies the simple, grounding and fundamental principles the words contain. Law professor Andrew Clapham believes that 'human rights are about each of us living in dignity,' and he goes on to point out that we are a long way from that being a reality. The movement that is needed to get us there, he believes, is one of 'people standing up to injustice and showing solidarity in the face of oppression.'[28]

Much like discussions of childbirth, talking about human rights tends to polarise discussion. On one side are those who believe they are a crucial tool in ensuring justice and dignity for all. An important way of navigating the needs, obligations and limitations of the individual within a bigger society. On the other side is a group who feel that the human rights movement privileges the dangerous and dishonourable at the expense of the innocent. Even that it binds our national legal systems in a way that makes life worse rather than better, or that it is the tool of criminals.

As you might imagine, I'm firmly in the first camp. Each of us as individuals has a special series of rights that we acquire by virtue of being human. The right to life, to freedom, not to be tortured, to be with our families, to have opinions and more. As individuals we desperately want these rights to be respected. Many of us take them for granted and, in the developed world at least, there is an innate expectation that these rights will be fulfilled. For life to be good for us, the vast majority of these rights must be protected.

Collectively human rights are a by-word for basic human dignity and say clearly to the state and the systems that it creates that individuals must be treated as human beings at all times and never as anything less. It's easy, by this definition, to begin to see why human rights could be a useful tool when approaching the complexities of reconciling the individual needs of women with the broader ambitions of society at large.

I see human rights as a self-supporting structure. We each want our own rights to be respected, but if our neighbour isn't treated with basic dignity the system begins to break down. When a neighbour's right to freedom is taken away arbitrarily the web becomes unstable. The more rights that are infringed the less protected my own are. I tend to illustrate this to school children with a giant Jenga tower, inviting them to pull a piece at a time as we gradually remove certain rights from entire groups of people. The bricks in the middle gradually become exposed. Eventually it becomes too unstable and the entire tower falls with a crash.

To me the human rights movement, the principles behind it and the various legal structures that contain it are trying to stop that crash. In order to do so the ideas have been translated into a series of formal agreements, treaties, covenants, international, regional and national laws and watchdogs. But beneath that formal framework we must remember that human rights are about protecting the essence of humanity in a complicated world.

The human rights legal framework

The beginnings of the formal human rights movement extend back to anti-slavery campaigning and some would argue even further. But the ideas as we recognise them today came to the fore in response to the atrocities of the Second World War. Genocide and war crimes represent to me the ultimate fall of the human rights Jenga tower, but the fall is previewed by the steady removal of other rights.

Throughout this book I choose to focus on three key human rights principles: dignity, autonomy and choice. These are the most relevant to childbirth and appear in different contexts throughout my arguments. On top of these principles sit the international, regional and domestic legal tools that codify and protect more explicit articulations of these ideas as concrete rights.

What follows is a brief, whistle-stop tour through the different layers of legal expression and protection of these rights. This tour is deliberately (for the sake of my own understanding and for purposes of brevity) over-simplified, but for those new to discussions of human rights it should give a basic understanding of the scaffolding around what many of us hold dear. For more see the Further Reading and Resources sections at the end of the book.

The Universal Declaration of Human Rights was adopted by the United Nations in 1948 and contains 30 articles detailing the extraordinary rights to which we are all entitled by virtue of being human. This rights blueprint is designed to help us navigate our life as individuals, interacting with the state and its representatives in a way that protects, addresses and privileges these rights – only suspending or removing them in thoughtful, specific and governed ways.

The rights in the Universal Declaration have since been co-opted into regional, national and international treaties and legal instruments. In 1976 the International Bill of Human Rights was ratified by enough nations to become international law. Preceding that, in September 1953, the European Convention on Human Rights came into effect. All Council of Europe members are party to it and any new member states are required to ratify it as soon as possible as a condition of joining. The Convention contains 18 articles and brought into being the European Court of Human Rights in 1959.

The Court, though not without its problems, acts as a court for the Council of Europe members. An individual, group of individuals or another state can bring a case against a state where it is believed they have violated one or more of the Articles in the European Convention. It's important to note (following the UK's EU referendum in June 2016) that membership of the European Union has no direct impact on our relationship to the European Court or Convention. These are not contingent on EU membership but on membership of the Council of Europe. While the post-Brexit rise in hate crimes acts as an all-too-real reminder of why human rights are important, there is no immediate threat to our current legal protections if the UK leaves the EU.

The UK and the Human Rights Act

Across the world states have taken human rights principles into their national legal framework to greater and lesser degrees. In the UK the Human Rights Act of 1998 (HRA) has taken 16 of the key rights from the European Convention on Human Rights and made them enforceable by law in the UK. This law sets out the minimum standards for how our government should behave towards us. The European Convention on Human Rights still applies to UK citizens, but most rights are more easily enforced using UK law. However, the European Court of Human Rights is still available and provides a higher authority if a case is unsuccessful in UK courts. These layers of protection for individuals should make it hard for the state to forget its obligations to us.

The HRA guarantees these minimum standards by placing a legal duty on public officials (including health services) to uphold these standards by respecting our human rights in everything they do. In addition all legislation, including health and social care law, should be compatible with human rights or 'human rights compliant'. In practice this means that the laws should be designed and applied in a way that respects, protects and fulfils our human rights. Though the HRA means public services and policies can be held to account as far as the courts, it is hoped that the act is mainly used to inform practice and policy to ensure legal action isn't needed.

As stated before, it's important to note, in the context of Britain's recent referendum on leaving the European Union, that Britain's relationship with the European Convention and Court would remain unchanged should they leave the EU, contingent as they are on membership of the Council of Europe.

Does this apply to me?

Public authorities and bodies exercising public functions have legal duties under the HRA. This includes: NHS organisations and staff (including commissioners), NHS services that have been outsourced to the the private sector or charities, local authorities and their employees including social services staff.

These duties apply regardless of your place on the hierarchy: from frontline practitioners like midwives, obstetricians and anaesthetists, to senior managers and board members.

Absolute, limited and qualified rights

Internationally states have different ways of balancing the rights of the individual against the broader needs of the state. In the UK rights fall into three different categories and are interpreted and enforced in different ways according to this.

Some rights are absolute. This means that they can never be taken away under any circumstances. Whatever the circumstances: the crime that someone may have committed, the information needed from them, the moral horror at what they've done or the unpopularity of their views, no one should ever be subjected to a violation of an absolute right. Because of this, absolute rights have a high threshold. Practically this means that something has to be very serious for it to qualify as a violation of an absolute right.

Article 3, the right to be free from inhuman and degrading treatment, is an absolute right and one that can and has been invoked in healthcare settings. After the failings at Mid-Staffordshire NHS Foundation Trust in England (including the labour ward), a public enquiry that resulted in the Francis Report of 2013 noted the terrible impact that a failure to respect dignity had on patients. To date over 100 successful human rights claims have been brought under Article 3 by former Mid-Staffordshire patients. Though the threshold is high for these claims, sadly violations can and do occur on this scale in the UK.

However, not all rights can be absolute if our society is to function well. Sometimes the rights of individuals directly conflict with the rights of others or society at large. In deference to this some rights are limited and can be restricted in specific circumstances. Article 5 – the right to liberty – is an obvious example. Individuals who have been convicted of a crime (after a fair trial and using appropriate procedure) can be imprisoned to protect others.

The final category of rights is 'qualified'. This qualification recognises that there is a need to balance the rights of the individual with the needs of the wider community or state. The right to private and family life (Article 8) is the right most often invoked around childbirth and is a qualified right.[29] A public authority can only interfere with a qualified right if it's allowed under the law. It must also show that it has a specific reason – as set out in the Human Rights Act – for interfering with your rights. These potential reasons are referred to as a 'legitimate aim' and include: the protection of health, the protection of other people's rights, the prevention of crime, national security and public safety. The interference must be no more than the minimum necessary to achieve one of the aims in the act.

Negative, positive and procedural duties

To protect you, the HRA says that those who have legal duties under it have three different kinds of duty. Negative duties mean they mustn't actively take away your rights, apart from in the specified circumstances we've discussed above.

Positive duties mean that public authorities must take positive action to protect rights. So if a group of people or an individual is in known danger of rights violations, the public body must do something to anticipate and mitigate that. In maternity care this could apply to vulnerable groups like disabled women, and a positive duty to think through their rights and protect them during their maternity care is placed on the systems and practitioners that care for these groups.

Procedural duties (though they sound a bit dull) are actually crucial to a well-functioning system. Public bodies must have systems in place to try to prevent abuses of human rights and properly investigate them if they do happen. Complaints procedures, inquests and the Parliamentary and Health Service Ombudsman should all be playing an active role in fulfilling the HRA's procedural duties in maternity care.

In addition to the legal framework, human rights principles are set out and reinforced in policy. An example of this is the health and social care regulator, the Care Quality Commission (CQC)'s policy, 'Human Rights Approach to the Regulation of Services'. This launched in September 2014 and now when the CQC inspects services – including maternity services – a human rights approach should be applied. The policy makes respectful maternity care a key part of the way healthcare benchmarks are set and measured.

This approach, along with other key professional standards and guideline documents that focus on maternity care (like the NICE Intrapartum Guidelines and the ambitions of the

National Maternity Review), increasingly privilege a human rights view through a focus on dignity, choice, consent and individual experience. The system itself and the culture around it are slower to do so. Legislation, policy and medical guidelines urgently need to be met with an infrastructure that actually allows midwives and doctors the chance to practise in a respectful way and offers them training on these approaches.

Outside the UK

Further afield international human rights law can and should have an impact on protecting citizens of almost all countries. Childbirth-related rights, invoking – as we will go on to discuss in more detail – some of the most fundamental and basic human rights, should be accessible to the majority of women across the world.

Though the Universal Declaration of Human Rights is not legally binding, it is used as an authoritative reference on – and has formed the basis for – international and national human rights instruments. At an international level these rights underpin the Universal Declaration and other declarations of the rights of specific groups and circumstances. A number of these declarations and covenants commit states to protecting and reporting on these rights. There is, however, no international court that focuses on broad human rights and therefore these international standards can be difficult to enforce if they are not strengthened by regional and national laws. The International Criminal Court (ICC), however, hears cases on genocide, war crimes and crimes against humanity. On 24 March 2016, 21 years after the massacre at Srebrenica and 12 years after my travels there, former Bosnian-Serb leader Radovan Karadžić was sentenced to 40 years in prison by the ICC for his leading role in the genocide.

Thankfully, regional protections are more tangibly

implemented. In addition to the European Convention, the African Charter on Human and Peoples' Rights for Africa of 1981 and the American Convention on Human Rights for the Americas of 1969 have been in force since 1986 and 1978 respectively.

The African Union and the Organization of American States perform a similar function in the human rights context to the Council of Europe. The Organization of American States covers north and south America, Canada and the Caribbean – 35 countries in total. The African Union covers almost all African states (54 in total) apart from Morocco, while Burkina Faso and the Central African Republic have currently suspended membership due to internal conflict. Each of these cross-border groups has documented specific rights in conventions and other legal documents and has created (or in the African Union's case is in the process of creating) a human rights court.

The common laws of most countries also protect some of the most fundamental rights that we are concerned with in this book. Increasingly, states have also incorporated explicit human rights articles in their domestic law – in a similar way to the Human Rights Act in the UK. In addition 110 countries have national human rights institutions to promote, monitor and protect human rights.

It is worth noting that Australia is an anomaly of sorts, not having a specific national 'bill of rights' like all other democratic countries. However, as a founding member of the United Nations, Australia is a signatory to the Universal Declaration of Human Rights and a number of the international treaties on human rights. The Australian Constitution protects key human rights and the Australian Human Rights Commission helps to monitor and safeguard them.

Collectively these structures should provide an increasingly robust system to ensure individuals are protected in a balanced way across the world. In real terms there are still huge challenges in enforcing human rights law – particularly in the developing world, but sadly all too often closer to home as well. Nevertheless, recent legal judgements from human rights courts are beginning to build layers of protection for pregnant and birthing women. Meanwhile, the principles that underpin the legislation are increasingly being used to influence culture and practice.

Childbirth in the international courtroom

In 2010 Anna Ternovszky challenged the state of Hungary at the European Court of Human Rights (ECHR) in a landmark case about a woman's right to choose the circumstances in which she gives birth. Remarkably, it was the first time the ECHR had considered a case related to childbirth and the impact of the judgement is still being felt. The case demonstrates how, in practical terms, international human rights instruments can be used to uphold, clarify and protect the rights of individuals.

Pregnant with her second baby, having had a previous homebirth with obstetrician-turned-midwife Ágnes Geréb, Ternovszky felt unable to plan another homebirth without challenging the law. Midwifery was not a recognised profession in Hungary and, as in a number of other countries, the legal status of homebirth was ambiguous. Midwives were unable to obtain the permits necessary to attend homebirths and, in the event of a poor outcome, automatically faced criminal prosecution rather than professional investigation. Geréb had previously had her licence to practise revoked for three years (following the death of a newborn) and was facing a manslaughter charge relating to another homebirth.

As Ternovszky passionately explains:

> *Out of fear that my second homebirth could trigger another case against my midwife, I turned to the ECHR to seek legal remedy. We accused the Hungarian state of violating two articles of the European Convention on Human Rights; one dealing with one's right to privacy and the other concerning its anti-discrimination regulation. The ECHR ruling was made within a year and found that both my rights had been violated.*

The Ternovszky case is no longer isolated, both in act and in remedy. Instead, it can be seen as part of an evolving approach to tackling childbirth issues that prioritises women's human rights, using that framework to push for change. In October 2014 the ECHR ruled on Konovalova v Russia, a case that reaffirmed that all decisions in childbirth require a woman's consent.

When Ms Konovalova gave birth in 1999 a large number of medical students crowded round her to observe, despite her express wish for them not to be present at this private moment. Russian courts found there was no legal requirement to seek consent for students' presence at a teaching hospital, so the case was taken to the ECHR, which ruled in Ms Konovalova's favour. The ruling stated that:

> *Article 8 encompasses the physical integrity of a person, since a person's body is the most intimate aspect of private life, and medical intervention, even if it is of minor importance, constitutes an interference with this right.*

Despite success at the European courts in both of these cases, progress has not continued unchecked. In December 2014 the

ECHR issued judgement on another homebirth-related case. The ruling in Dubská v Czech Republic, seen by many as an important successor to the Ternovszky case, was expected to further underline a woman's right to choose where to give birth. But in a move that has shocked and concerned human rights experts and campaigners, the court ruled in the opposite direction; it decided that prohibiting midwives from attending homebirths in the Czech Republic did not contravene women's human rights.

Human rights barrister and founder of Birthrights, Elizabeth Prochaska, expresses concern that such contradictory judgements are a risk to the credibility of the ECHR. It is hard to understand how different sections of the same court could come to such inconsistent judgements as Ternovszky and Dubská. It was frighteningly clear during the Dubská case that within the Czech hospital system much was at fault. The United Nations[30] has condemned the care Czech women receive in hospital and the court heard of human rights violations, forced medical procedures and mandatory in-hospital monitoring for 72 hours after birth. Despite accepting the evidence on the safety of homebirth (from large-scale studies like Birthplace in England[31]), it seems that testimony from a Czech obstetrician on the dangers of 'unexpected difficulties' that could be faced by babies at a homebirth played a significant part in the court's decision-making.

Although the judges noted explicitly that 'power struggles' between midwives and doctors were at work in the homebirth debate in the Czech Republic, Prochaska believes the court fell into the 'age-old mistake of preferring a personal account (by a doctor implicated in the "power struggle") over tested evidence of risk'. Aside from risk debates, however flawed, it is worrying that a human rights court is privileging medical opinion over an individual's freedom to access the care that they believe is safest and most appropriate for them. Czech women who wish to avoid the dangers within the hospital system are, for now, forced to give birth without medical assistance or to find a midwife prepared to practise illegally and face possible imprisonment.[32]

The Grand Chamber of the court has subsequently heard an appeal in the Dubská case and the judgement is long-awaited. It is hoped that the Grand Chamber will ensure the final judgement in Dubská upholds women's rights in the birth room. As more and more legal challenges around childbirth appear in the ECHR pipeline there is still much hope. A fourth case, Cypiene v Lithuania, which also focuses on a right to choose one's place of birth, is awaiting a decision after the Dubská appeal.

Although these rulings mean a great deal to women and those who care for them, the personal dangers to midwives who attend homebirths are slow to recede. Despite the 2010 ECHR victory, Ternovszky's midwife Ágnes Geréb was later imprisoned and spent over three years under house arrest following a negligence conviction related to homebirths. Her investigation and trial have been heavily criticised. Donal Kerry of the 'Justice for Dr Geréb Movement' explains that double standards mean that Geréb, who has recorded over 3,500 healthy homebirths, with only three fatalities in 17 years, faced automatic criminal investigation for any poor outcome, while 'hospital adverse incidents are first investigated by their professional peers and rarely, if ever, get referred to the police for criminal investigation.'

Geréb's house arrest was lifted in February 2014, but she is forbidden to leave Hungary and the 10-year suspension of her medical licence remains in force. In July 2014, the Capital Court of Appeal announced an investigation that could lead to a retrial. It remains impossible for a midwife to get a fair trial in Hungary: biased and inappropriately qualified expert witnesses are allowed to give their opinions, but midwives and international homebirth experts are not registered on the courts' current expert list and cannot therefore be called as witnesses.

There are five current cases against Agnes Geréb and she continues to be processed through the criminal court with no certainty in the outcome. In October 2015 a campaign was started to raise the €11,800 needed to meet legal and medical fees connected with her court cases. It took less than a month for the campaign to reach its target.

The human rights legal framework is providing a powerful way to challenge states that don't protect the rights of pregnant women, but it will take time, investment and training for the positive implications to be felt by all women and healthcare professionals, particularly if backward steps like the Dubská judgement are thrown in the way. In the UK, applying this approach to maternity care is slowly becoming more common at an individual practitioner, institution and policy level. Dr Amali Lokugamage, an author and consultant obstetrician, explains that in her clinical practice she is very aware of women's autonomy and bodily integrity. She adds that she doesn't 'feel challenged or unsettled or upset' when her advice is not taken, because she recognises that a woman has authority. She is using human rights tools explicitly in her education of postgraduate students and fellows of the Royal College of Obstetricians and Gynaecologists to positive effect.

Yet Lokugamage admits that her style is far from the norm. Most obstetricians have a lack of training in human or civil rights and find it harder to retain the same sensitivity, particularly if a woman wishes to pursue something against their recommendation. Explaining their discomfort, she describes a 'litigation atmosphere in obstetrics', where fear of negligence claims leads healthcare professionals to defensive practice. Although she feels confident that mandatory training in human rights would go a long way to rectifying this, she explains that in an underfunded service it is difficult to prioritise.

As well as not promoting a rights-based approach, the culture within obstetric training could be contributing to the problem. In a 2014 survey by the UK's General Medical Council,[33] trainees in the obstetrics and gynaecology speciality were the most likely to have experienced bullying and undermining within the profession. In a study of obstetric and gynaecology consultants in 2016[34] 44 per cent reported that they had been persistently bullied or undermined. Midwives also report high levels of bullying and stress-related sick leave and a recent Royal College of Midwives report[35] showed that 46 per cent of midwives surveyed were experiencing high levels of work-related stress. That those who are trained and work in a system that overworks, undermines and bullies them aren't espousing an individualised, compassionate approach is hardly surprising.

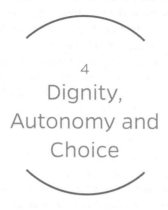

4
Dignity, Autonomy and Choice

Dignity

The label and framework of human rights may be relatively new in the childbirth arena, but one of its key concepts, 'dignity', has become a buzzword in healthcare settings. An initial focus on dignity in end-of-life care has spread outwards, and the UK's National Dignity Council has over 50,000 'Dignity Champions' in place, raising awareness of respectful care and modelling good practice. Looking at dignity not simply as an approach to improving the experience of care, but as an antidote to unsafe practice, has become popular since the 2013 publication of Robert Francis's inquiry into failings at Mid-Staffordshire NHS Trust. Francis identified disrespectful and abusive care as central to the issues. In response, the UK's Department of Health prioritised the inclusion of 'basic values of dignity and respect' in training for healthcare professionals.

So what is 'dignity' and, when applied to childbirth, can it mean more than the idea that we leave our dignity at the door? Human rights barrister Elizabeth Prochaska thinks so and cites Kant's categorical imperative that 'a person should be treated as an end and not a means'[36] by way of explanation. Although giving birth may at times not be 'dignified' in itself, affording a labouring woman dignity means respecting her humanity despite her pregnant status. Prochaska describes this imperative as 'particularly powerful' in the maternity context, where a woman is commonly treated as the means for the production of a baby, rather than an end in herself. In this scenario her interests are often 'diminished or neglected in preference for the baby's'.

Professor of psychiatry Harvey Chochinov is an expert in the idea of 'dignity' and takes this idea further. In his eyes the respect that needs to be afforded to women at this time is magnified by the physical, mental and emotional challenges of labour or surgery. These may render her more vulnerable and less capable of asserting herself than usual. Chochinov suggests that childbirth itself can take a toll on women's autonomy 'by way of yielding to the will of their bodies', and that this can lead to a presumption that they are no longer whole or worthwhile persons. He challenges that assumption, stating that 'giving birth makes one no less a person' and reminding us that vulnerability is part of the essence of what it means to be human.

In Chochinov's eyes, when a person's natural autonomy is weakened, perhaps during childbirth, if outside forces make a woman feel weak, inadequate and otherwise undermine her sense of dignity, she 'will feel the assault of these harsh judgements and may internalise them as being reflective of her self-worth'. Chochinov's explanation fits neatly with evidence showing that many women who experience childbirth negatively report a profound impact on how they feel about themselves.

Thankfully, it's clear from a number of recent surveys and

pieces of research that the majority of British women feel they have received broadly dignified, kind and compassionate care from their midwives and doctors during childbirth. In the 2013 Birthrights survey, 82 per cent of women noted that they felt respected by midwives and medical staff. However, within that overall satisfaction there are pockets of concern, with a quarter of women in London, and a quarter of those who had instrumental births, not feeling their care was respectful.

Across the world the variations in care are as dramatic as the systems, or lack of systems, that contain them. The 2014 statement by the World Health Organization (WHO) on the prevention and elimination of disrespect and abuse during childbirth reports that abusive treatment during childbirth has included outright physical abuse,[37] profound humiliation and verbal abuse. A study reported in *The Lancet* analysed human rights violations in maternity care, characterising them as often deliberate and related to poor-quality healthcare services. The study authors went on to add that this abuse is a system used to control patients and that it is learnt and reinforced in health facilities.[38]

I believe that dignity principles provide a remedy to this, in both the developed and developing world, and can act against rights abuses and sub-standard care across the spectrum of severity. When dignity is missing from maternity care the impact on individuals is profound.

A lonely machine

Michaelis[39] lives in the remote Indigenous Australian community of Saint Gerard, in the Northern Territory. When she had her first baby, like every woman across every single remote community in Australia, she had no birth options. Evacuated by air, weeks before her due date, she was sent 500km to Darwin to wait alone in a hostel for labour to begin.

Fellow Saint Gerard resident Theodora described the hostel as full 'of people humbugging you for money and drunks making you scared'. Other hostel residents have described a lack of food and threats of gang violence.

It is no secret that the Australia-wide practice of removing this particularly vulnerable group of women from their communities, often against their wishes, at a personally and culturally significant time, isn't working. Yet the only options open to Indigenous Australian women to avoid it are to opt out of care altogether, or go to a local clinic so late in labour that they cannot be transferred. Even then, routine practice is to stop a low-risk, full-term, well-progressing labour with drugs and airlift the mother to Darwin. A birth that has been interrupted by drugs and transfer may be difficult to restart without the use of significant intervention, with potential for serious impact on mother and baby.

Australian policy documents from as early as the 1980s express the need for birth facilities for women in their local communities. The recent five-year National Maternity Services Plan[40] sets out a timetable for introducing birthing 'on country' programmes for Aboriginal and Torres Strait Islander women. Although research has been carried out, and indigenous women from every state and every territory flocked to a recent national workshop, there is currently no government funding for services that the plan promised would be ready last year. Currently, not a single scheme exists in Australia to provide 'on country' birthing in remote areas.

Michaelis was upset by what she experienced in the city, far away from her family. 'When I had the baby, there were big mobs of people and male doctors watching. I was on the bed and told to open my legs up. I didn't like being there, I didn't like the men being there and I didn't like being watched. It was such a shame job.'[41]

Aboriginal and Torres Strait Islanders' lives are based around a complex series of beliefs, rituals and rights, all deeply connected to the wider idea of the Dreaming. Men and women often have separate ceremonies, with different sacred objects. They are seen as guardians of distinct sections of folk law and community knowledge, sometimes referred to as the laws of women's or men's 'business'. Birth, or 'borning', falls inevitably within the women's business laws. The indigenous people of Australia are not a homogenous group, and their rituals and practices around birth differ across communities. Nevertheless, pregnancy and birth are viewed across the board as a significant rite of passage; not only for the new spirit (who, it is often believed, will enter the foetus in the fifth month of pregnancy), but also for the woman herself and those around her.

Men are traditionally not part of the process and many women report shame at giving birth in their presence. Aunties and other female members of the community traditionally gather to give massage and practical support to a woman as she labours.

It is hard for those of us outside the Indigenous Australian community to begin to understand the importance for them that their infants are born in their home territory. Midwifery professor Hannah Dahlen explains that there are groups who believe a child's spirit will weaken and it will die if it is not born on the land. Without the vocabulary to describe the relationship, we are grasping at comparisons that don't really do it justice. Nala Mansell-McKenna, a youth worker, explains the difference, as he sees it, between indigenous and non-indigenous approaches to land: 'In white society, a person's home is a structure made of bricks or timber, but to our people our home was the land that we hunted and gathered on and held ceremony.'[42] More simply, Natasha Neidje describes her feelings for her country as 'like the love for your mum and dad'.[43]

Much is becoming known about the process of removing indigenous peoples from their country, the separation of their children, the part-destruction of their heritage and the catastrophic effect it has had on the generations that followed. That effect is shown to ripple out across health outcomes. Indigenous Australians live approximately 20 years less than the rest of the population. Maternal mortality is 3.5 times higher among Aboriginal and Torres Strait Islander people, and their babies are more than twice as likely to die after birth.

Francesca, mother to many children, was also evacuated from Saint Gerard to Darwin to have some of her babies. She missed the support of the community and felt exposed and alone. 'It takes a long time [labour], always them watching, and they put you on to a lonely machine; no company, no one to rub you, just a green bowl and cold water to wash your face in.'

At the end of her busy spring day and the beginning of my autumn one, I talk to Professor Sue Kildea, an Australian midwife and researcher who has worked extensively within indigenous communities. She angrily explains that there has never been an official policy on what facilities should be provided to remote communities for birth, but that as rural birth centres and services have been subject to 'unbelievable closures' across Australia, removing women to the nearest large-scale obstetric unit has become the default. She cites a key motivation as being an attempt to deal with previously high rates of perinatal mortality, but also stresses that evacuation of remote women is tied up in what she describes as 'the fear and medicalisation of birth that's pretty rife in Australia'.

Although the practice may have originally had good intentions, Kildea believes its blanket application in the face of contemporary knowledge is 'horrible and dreadful'. She describes how women can be away for weeks, at a really

important time in their lives, and are lonely and isolated.
She adds:

> It was never really a choice. Women were just told
> they couldn't have their babies where they wanted and
> that they couldn't take a relative with them to the city.
> That's still what happens today. They acquiesce because
> they don't perceive that they have a choice. In all of the
> projects that talk to women about what they want, the
> message is the same. What we are doing at the moment
> is not considered culturally safe for women. They are
> desperately worried and it's extraordinary that we still
> get it so wrong on almost every level.

Michaelis's experiences in Darwin meant that in future
she avoided evacuation by staying away from antenatal care
– 'Don't talk about it. Sit down quiet until it's ready'. Mary
Magdalene believed that if her pregnancy was found out she
would be sent to Darwin against her will, so she chose to
keep it secret. 'I wanted to have this one here in Saint Gerard
and keep it watmam [quiet] from everyone. I didn't want the
nurses to know the plan because I was scared they would send
me to Darwin anyway.'

The lack of cultural safety prompted these women to give
birth in a local setting, even though there are no birthing
facilities provided for them. Without these facilities it is hard
to view their decisions as free choice. While only a minority
of indigenous women choose to stay at home, as Kildea points
out, 'If one in ten of the women in my caseload are avoiding
the system, even though they are committed to doing what
they think is safest for their babies and, as a culture, are very
adaptable, the system is not working.'

By contrast, the Canadian Inuit people, who have faced

similar challenges and whose belief about the importance of birthing in community is comparable, have slowly brought birth back over the past 30 years. In response to a series of suicides of young people, elder women from Nunavik opened a birth centre in this remote area, far away from access to obstetric facilities.

Despite outside concerns about safety, excellent outcomes for both mother and baby have been shown across a number of studies,[44] and community birth for remote Inuit people is becoming the norm. The impact has been broader than expected, with research showing a drop in domestic violence in areas where mothers were no longer evacuated for birth.

Back in Australia, Kildea is thoughtful about the importance of where babies are born to indigenous communities. 'Everyone in those remote communities knows which babies have been born there and which ones haven't. It's different and we simply can't measure the strength and resilience that comes from that community birth in a Western framework.'

Kildea's mentor, award-winning health worker Molly Wardaguga (now deceased), felt that the dysfunction of the Indigenous Australian community was directly attributable to the way babies were being born. In a community with increasing mental health problems, high suicide rates, high rates of drug and alcohol abuse as well as unemployment, it is hard to ignore the dislocation that happens at the start of life. What is bad for women is bad for their babies and the community at large.

Yet, despite examples from Canada and New Zealand demonstrating that birth 'on country' can be safe and deliverable, change is not happening. The ability of women to exercise their basic right to choose where and with whom to give birth, as affirmed by the ECHR's Ternovszky ruling, is seemingly impossible to promote for those who are almost voiceless. Kildea relates the struggle to the wider problem of women's place in society and the lack of importance attributed to them. She cites a pandemic of institutional racism working in tandem with a patriarchal obstetric system as key factors preventing progress on the issue.

When consideration for their wider cultural safety and basic human dignity is missing from the systems in which people give birth, much is lost. Though most prominently and profoundly affecting those women made vulnerable by their indigenous status, the lack of regard for women's right to choose begins to be felt by others. Access to homebirth across Australia has met with strong opposition, particularly from the private obstetric lobby, which has a financial incentive to make sure it doesn't succeed. In 2009 it very nearly became effectively illegal, with insurance requirements for independent midwives being impossible to fulfil and no state-sponsored homebirth service available. Protests secured an exemption to the insurance requirements. This exemption has been extended, but there has been no definitive resolution.

Despite compelling evidence demonstrating the safety of homebirth, its cost-effectiveness and capacity to reduce interventions and improve maternal satisfaction (particularly via the UK's 2011 Birthplace in England study[45] of around 70,000 women), the Australian obstetric umbrella organisation, RANZCOG, has its fingers firmly in its ears. Its statement on the subject misleadingly asserts that 'no studies are available to evaluate the cost-effectiveness of homebirth in comparison to birth in other settings'.[46] It does not support planned homebirth.

The inhumane approach to remote childbirth in indigenous communities across Australia shows the cost to individuals when dignity is absented from their care. Though RANZCOG insists that it 'strongly supports' considering the wishes of all women in decisions about birth, it shies away from actually recommending any tangible 'on country' birth options. Without healthcare structures in place offering meaningful choice and access to physically and culturally safe care for all women, support is merely rhetorical. Be it for low-risk Indigenous Australian women unwilling to get on that plane, or others keen to exercise their right to choose where they give birth: if women's wishes are missing from the picture the prevailing order is not working.

Caregivers and autonomy: whose decision is it anyway?

In 2013 midwives and obstetricians were asked to rate their agreement with the statement: '*The final decision should always rest with the woman.*'[47] The vast majority agreed. They were then asked whether they agreed with a contradictory statement: '*For the safety of the baby, the maternity care team sometimes needs to override the needs of the woman.*' A large number of those who had felt that decision-making should rest with the woman later agreed that her needs could be overridden for the sake of her baby.

Their confused thinking is understandable. It is challenging and uncomfortable to accept that if we respect women's autonomy in pregnancy, they may not always make what we consider to be the right decisions for their baby. In many legal systems rights aren't conferred on a foetus until the woman, who has been nurturing it, gives birth. This doesn't prevent us from seeing a baby from the very start and wanting to protect it.

How best to do that is a question that sparks the above confusion, and at the heart of that is how we conceptualise the relationship between a mother and foetus. Much has been made by the anti-abortion movement of the fact that an unborn baby is not simply another part of the mother before birth. In addition, as Clare Murphy of the British

Pregnancy Advisory Service (bpas) notes, 'increasingly public health efforts seem focused on protecting foetuses from their mother's behaviour'. We are often encouraged to see mothers and foetuses as separate and competing entities, when the reality is far more complex. An analysis concluding that a woman and the baby she is carrying in her womb are the same being, or indeed one that suggests that they are two wholly different, competing beings, is too simple and flawed.

I prefer the idea of the mother/foetus relationship as the result of an involuntary, biological process and thus 'unique amongst human relations'.[48] Here the woman and foetus are characterised as 'separate but symbiotic organisms bonded in a union separable only by birth'. Attempts to pit mother and foetus against each other antagonistically are belied by the physical realities of pregnancy. Crucially, a pregnant woman nourishes and sustains the foetus inside her womb, with all the risks to her own health and life that that brings with it. Truly, women and the babies growing inside them are neither separate, nor one and the same. They are distinct, but cannot be separated conceptually.

UK court records from the past 20 years demonstrate the problems with viewing mother and foetus as in competition. In the late 1990s, S was diagnosed with pre-eclampsia but decided against the recommended induction. Although she was deemed competent to make decisions and was not suffering from serious mental illness, she was detained under the Mental Health Act. A judge allowed her consent to be overridden and against her express wishes she was operated on and her baby was born by caesarean. Later, the Appeal Court held that S's right to autonomy had been violated and that her detention had been against the law. The courts upheld that a competent pregnant woman could refuse treatment even if that refusal might result in harm to her or her unborn child.

Again, this decision and the stark choices it appears to paint can seem difficult for many of us to accept. Should we be allowing women to make choices that aren't in the best interests of the baby? I say categorically yes, with the reassurance that the overwhelming majority of mothers are trying to make choices during pregnancy and birth that are good for their babies. It feels uncomfortable to accept that occasionally maternal autonomy may result in a poor outcome for the baby. But there is no one else better placed or better motivated to make a positive decision for the unborn child.

If we take away maternal autonomy, to whom do we give decision-making power? How do we ensure that these decisions are unbiased and backed by the best evidence? Looking at the differences in obstetric practice between seemingly comparable countries like the UK, Italy and America, who on earth would we credit with truly knowing what is best? There is no objective view. English courts have repeatedly asserted that women have to be trusted to make their own decisions, even if they go against medical opinion. Occasionally, women will get it wrong, just as sometimes medical professionals do. There is no childbirth without risk, though risks are usually small in the developed world. Given access to honest information, evidence and good support, women can interpret and choose risks for themselves and their babies. For some, the lowest risk on paper may not be the best option. Unless a woman is genuinely mentally incapable of making an informed decision, I believe that overall the safest outcomes are when women are the ones with the final say. There is no choice to be made between woman and foetus. There is no competition. We must support the woman to make the choices she needs to for them both in good faith.

The case of Laura Pemberton, an American woman pregnant with her second baby, exemplifies what's at stake when the state takes control. After a previous caesarean, Laura's obstetrician had refused to allow her to attempt the vaginal birth she desperately wanted. While UK women are usually advised to attempt a vaginal birth after a previous caesarean, most US obstetricians will insist on the opposite. Laura Pemberton's only option, if she wanted to attempt birth in the way she believed was best for her and her baby, was a homebirth with a private midwife.

While in labour she tried to go to hospital, needing a drip for rehydration. Instead, she was refused treatment until she signed consent for a caesarean. Desperate to avoid this unless it was actually necessary, she ran barefoot from the hospital, still in active labour. At home, examinations by her midwife showed progress was being made and mother and baby were doing well.

Later, a knock on the door disturbed her peaceful labouring. A deputy sheriff and state attorney stood on the doorstep and informed her that they had a court order allowing them to transport her to hospital and operate on her. Laura began hysterically pleading with the state attorney not to take her in.

Humiliated and terrified, she was strapped to a stretcher and put in the back of an ambulance, her previously steady blood pressure rising as she travelled. As she changed into her hospital gown she could feel the top of the baby's head coming down, and in desperation she pushed and tried to reach in and pull the baby out, to 'prevent them from taking it the way they wanted to'.

In a final examination before surgery she was found to be nine centimetres dilated; nearly ready to give birth without intervention. With mother and unborn baby in good health, she asked again to be allowed to try but was informed that her baby was in the control of the state which was responsible for it. The surgeon made the cut and the baby was born by caesarean section. Laura says she feels she has 'been raped by the system'.

A later suit against the hospital was dismissed, the courts asserting that the caesarean was deemed to be necessary by doctors to avoid substantial risk that the baby would die during delivery. It affirmed that the state's interest in preserving the life of an unborn child outweighed the mother's constitutional interest of bodily integrity. The mother's own perception of risk and benefit, which appears more closely tied to the reality of the situation, was regarded as worthless.[49]

Since Laura's case, US legislators increasingly appear to be buying into the flawed idea of mother and foetus acting in competition, with mothers disappearing from view in discussions of pregnancy and birth. Even where the law takes a more humane view, confusion abounds as to how to handle situations where medical opinion disagrees with women's wishes, or where practices that might be culturally safe and preferable for mothers are not understood or made possible by infrastructure.

A significant portion of US hospitals and obstetricians operate a 'VBAC ban' – refusing to care for women who request a vaginal birth after a caesarean section. Dr Stuart Fishbein, a Californian obstetrician/gynaecologist, is clear that this policy is in conflict with doctors' code of ethics and basic standards of care.

> *Every obstetrician and hospital administrator who isn't vehemently opposing their facilities VBAC ban is violating the code of ethics they swore to uphold. Every obstetrician who doesn't support the reasonable option of VBAC by either offering it or referring to someone who does is practicing beneath the standard of care. A system that continues to allow these people to direct programs*

and allows them to maintain positions of authority is a flawed system. That's reality. Let's be honest.

Viewing mothers and foetuses as distinct but intrinsically connected allows us to realise that their interests are not separate and competing, but complex, interlinked and interdependent. The next logical step is to accept the legal position in many countries that places decision-making entirely in the remit of the mother, acknowledging that the overwhelming majority will act in accordance with the additional responsibility that their pregnancy has placed on them and providing social remedy in the rare cases where they don't.

There are no sides to take in this argument. A person and the baby they grow are served best when they are allowed to make their own decisions with appropriate supportive care if desired and evidence-based information. Trusting them to do the right thing for their family, and making the system around them underpin that, will be far more effective in improving the baby's future. The myth of the 'bad mother' should be stamped on. The tiny sliver of truth that it contains is best dealt with individually, not by presuming all women are inherently dangerous to their babies and trying to coerce or force them to be compliant.

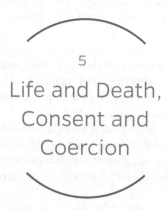

5

Life and Death, Consent and Coercion

Survival and respect

Rahema[50] arrived at Meru District Hospital in rural Tanzania at the end of the midwives' nine-hour shift. She was already beginning to push her baby out. When Camella (a UK midwife working on the ward) was able to get to her, she saw that the baby was in the breech position. Staff gathered round. Just as the baby was descending, the electricity cut out and everything was plunged into darkness. The only light available was a bike lamp from her pocket which flashed intermittently. In the occasional burst of light Camella saw the tiny baby was in poor condition and skilfully resuscitated her. Suddenly, she saw signs that another baby was about to be born. An overwhelmed Rahema, who had struggled with the Tanzanian taboo of infertility for 10 years, was mother to unexpected twins. Just as she began to realise that she had not one but two live babies, Rahema started to lose blood at a frightening pace. Camella had to stitch her swiftly, but without drugs to stop the bleeding she would die. Rahema did not have the funds to pay for the drugs, so the midwife paid for them herself. Without her, Rahema would have bled to death then and there, her newborn twins would have become newborn orphans and Rahema another statistic.

To ensure that basic rights are upheld throughout pregnancy and birth, legal principles (that all healthcare professionals should respect) are codified to some degree in law in every country in the world. As human rights barrister Elizabeth Prochaska notes, 'on paper, all countries respect women's right to consent to treatment and to be treated without discrimination.'

Article 25 of the Universal Declaration of Human Rights asserts a right to an adequate standard of healthcare and additional special protection for mothers and children. Yet according to WHO, 800 women die every day from preventable causes and 99 per cent of those are in the developing world. While maternal mortality has reduced by 50 per cent since 1990, the UN's pledge to cut 75 per cent of maternal deaths by 2015 was the millennium development goal furthest off target. Between 2016 and 2030, as part of the Sustainable Development Agenda, the new target is to reduce the global maternal mortality ratio to less than 70 per 100,000 live births. Today more than half of maternal deaths occur in sub-Saharan Africa and almost one-third in South Asia. The maternal mortality ratio in developing countries in 2013 was 230 per 100,000 live births, versus 16 in developed countries. The disparity here is shocking and its effects are profound.

For most Tanzanian citizens poverty remains a reality. Women in rural areas have on average 6.1 children and WHO estimates that maternal mortality is as high as 410 women per 100,000 births. Camella Main (the UK midwife working in rural Tanzania who caught Rahema's twins) describes Meru District Hospital, making it clear what a difficult place Tanzania is for birthing women and how far they are from being able to access adequate healthcare.

'There's no running water and only intermittent electricity,' she says, detailing poor sanitation, filthy buildings where women must share a bed, failings in infection control and no water to drink. 'Mosquitos are rife and malaria thrives,' she adds. 'The labour ward has only dirty utensils for carrying out suturing and when there are no clamps we tie the baby's cord with string.'

Not allowed in from the courtyard until a baby's head is visible, women have only thin mattresses on which to give birth. Despite women's preferences, and evidence suggesting dynamic positions are optimal for birth, here obstetric ritual dictates that women must lie completely flat to give birth. This position makes it hard to push, more difficult for the baby to navigate through the pelvis and is often far more painful. Once their babies arrive, new mothers can stay on the overcrowded postnatal wards, where they receive no care, but can at least rest before they walk many miles home with or without their newborns.

For Tanzanian women, safe maternity care can't be guaranteed without the chance to give birth with dignity, compassion and respect. Since talking to Camella about her time in Tanzania I've had the opportunity to see conditions in some areas for myself. In February 2016 I visited the Shinyanga region as a guest of Amref Health Africa, a leading health charity. Accompanied by their team I travelled from the capital Dar Es Salaam to some of the most remote villages in the north of this beautiful but troubled country.

Amref's projects have upgraded the local health centres from the dirty, under-staffed and sometimes abusive places that Camella describes. The conditions are still basic, but the health centres I visited at Uteshu and Masumbwe were impeccably clean, filled with seemingly well-trained staff, equipped with autoclaves for sterilising equipment and ambulances to transport those in difficulty. Most importantly perhaps for women was the additional obstetric training and facilities, meaning that caesarean sections, tubal ligation (female sterilisation) and other vital operative services were now provided.

With four in ten women getting married before the age of 18, and the average age of first birth being 19, young women will get to know these facilities well. For those who are lucky to live close to an Amref project they can expect safe and respectful care, as well as access to family planning, HIV clinics and sexual health education – though only if their husbands or fathers-in-law will allow them to take advantage of the facilities. But the women of a village called Lunguya told me what it was like to live a six- to seven-hour walk from their local health centre. Even this comparatively short distance from the facilities can be a matter of life and death, and they are campaigning for a local dispensary so that healthy women without complications can give birth closer to home.

The drive to get women to give birth away from their homes and traditional practices and in centralised health centres is one that gives me some unease – especially now that we see the imperfect aftermath of the same drive here in the UK. In the context of stories from indigenous women in Australia, and the emerging evidence about the importance of environment in labour, I have found it hard to reconcile the banning of traditional birth attendants in Tanzania and other countries with my knowledge of the value women place on non-clinical support in labour and birth.

Speaking to women and seeing the infrastructure has helped a little. And while it should be a clear goal to ensure that women have facilities close to home and continuity of carer, the current challenge is simply providing safe, accessible basic facilities and education. The women I talked to were positive about birthing at the health centres, seeing them as places of sanctuary and hope, particularly because of the family planning and HIV clinics. Education programmes appeared collaborative and not coercive – perhaps why they were so successful – and crucially an environment of respect was present at all the facilities I visited.

Thirty-year-old Paskazia Amos, a nurse and midwife at Masumbwe health centre, explained how the facilities have developed in recent years and just what is at stake, given the lack of transport, infrastructure and training in some areas.

Before Masumbwe Health Centre was upgraded, women and babies were dying who we could have saved given the facilities. The staff knew it and I think the women knew it too. One night a woman came who was deep in labour. It wasn't going well – there were too many complications for us to handle. We simply didn't have the equipment and training. So the doctors agreed we should refer her to the district hospital. It felt like a death sentence for her and she seemed to know it.

When I told her she had to transfer she kept crying and saying 'Don't send me there, I will die.' It was a long journey and they were so busy when she arrived that it took them more than six hours to take her to theatre. Then she bled to death on the table. Now when I see her husband I feel terrible. I wish we could have saved her. If she had come to us today she wouldn't have died. It's hard to live with but I can't change it. Now I focus on preventing that happening again.

With the additional training from the Amref project I'm now a specialist anaesthetic nurse. Last week I was attending to a woman having a caesarean and training a student in the procedure. A junior nurse came to tell me that a woman had arrived with a stillborn breech baby.

It's sometimes hard to know where to go, how to split yourself between the people who need you.

Even though I had to make difficult decisions that night I'm proud of how I handled it. I was able to leave my student with the doctors in the caesarean. I went to the labouring woman and confirmed that her baby had died. It's never easy to tell people terrible truths but I was able to spend some time with her giving comfort. Then I helped her birth her dead baby and stopped her haemorrhaging. I was able to return to supervise a difficult part of the caesarean. We saved two women and a baby in very complex circumstances in the space of minutes that night. It's not always easy but it's worth it.

At Uteshu health centre, some four hours' drive away, Dr Nicodemus Senguo explained that they were wildly exceeding their expected quota of patients every month. Having heard about the good facilities, the adequate staffing and respectful approach, people are travelling up to 70km to be treated there. When provided with culturally sensitive, respectful care that is saving the lives of women and their babies, communities vote with their feet.

Brigid McConville, UK director of the White Ribbon Alliance, explains that respectful care is one of the life and death issues in the developing world 'because if women hear bad reports from others and fear they will be abused at a health centre, they simply won't go'. Pointing to what some have called 'ghost hospitals' in some countries in sub-Saharan Africa (staffed and equipped but largely deserted), she adds that evidence is now emerging that respectful care could be even more important in saving mothers' lives than issues of transport or cost. Far from being the icing on the cake, care that prioritises dignity encourages women to use a service that could save their lives.

When women can expect physical and emotional abuse in places of theoretical safety, it is unsurprising that they are unwilling to change established cultural practice around birth and use a hospital or trained birth attendant during labour. On Camella Main's first day in Tanzania she witnessed a midwife and doctor slapping and pinching a 16-year-old girl who was making noise to cope with her contractions. She describes it as 'extremely distressing to witness and even harder to stop'.

Inequalities of and in birth

It is not simply a lack of access to care, or inadequate care and abusive practices, that women in the developing world face. A 2006 report from Human Rights Watch (HRW), a non-governmental organisation (NGO), highlighted the plight of those who, faced with complex pregnancies, need to seek obstetric care during childbirth. Unable to pay their medical bills, they are detained indefinitely after the birth; frequently without adequate food and in overcrowded conditions.

An 18-year-old woman, being held at Prince Louis Rwagasore Clinic, Burundi, was interviewed by HRW: 'I had to come to hospital because I needed a caesarean. When I got the bill, the doctor said to me, "Since you have not paid, we will keep you here." I don't have permission to leave with my baby. We are often hungry here. I cannot stand this situation any longer.'[51]

Burundi is party to a number of international human rights covenants that are violated by this kind of forced detention in inhumane conditions. They are also obliged under these to work towards a better standard of health; something that is perhaps prompting progress. In 2006, Burundi took a step towards those obligations with a presidential order on maternal and child healthcare, promising free care to child-bearing women. Yet the practice of detention of other patients, corruption and lack of investment in healthcare, remain a reality for Burundians today.

Problems such as these are not limited to Burundi. In many areas of the developing world, women with difficult labours rely on the goodwill of doctors or a benefactor who can cover their medical bills. Those unable to do so risk becoming part of what WHO calls 'unacceptably high' maternal mortality rates. Numbers of women imprisoned after hospital treatment during childbirth are impossible to come by, but detention is still rife in a number of countries, including Zimbabwe, Liberia, the Philippines and Kenya.

The inability to pay for care may not lead directly to imprisonment in the developed world, but finance has been tightly linked to the deaths of mothers and babies in the US. WHO enumerates a need for the US 'to look at improving access to the most marginalised individuals', listing 'women in rural areas, those of lower socioeconomic status, minority ethnic groups, and those without health insurance' as liable to have difficulty accessing care.

Thankfully, the recent Affordable Health Care for America Act means that all health insurance policies are now required to cover maternity care. However, undocumented people above the Medicaid cut-off, those who are afraid to enrol in Medicaid and people who have not purchased private insurance find themselves without maternity care. Those who have insurance may find it funnels them towards a care pathway that they believe is unsafe for them or their babies. In many ways comparable with the indigenous women of Australia's remote communities, some American women who are keen to avoid unnecessary intervention in childbirth can only do so if they give birth at home without any clinical care. In one international social media group offering support to women planning unassisted childbirth, a number of US women confirmed that their intention to give birth without a midwife or doctor present stemmed initially from their insurance not covering midwife-led care or homebirth. Unwilling to submit to obstetric practices that they believed were harmful for their own or their baby's wellbeing, unassisted birth was their only option. Unassisted childbirth can be a positive and informed choice that (certainly in the UK) is within a woman's legal right to make. I will discuss this later on. However, the inability to pay for care, or pay for care in the birth setting of a woman's choice, as well as anxiety about paying for emergency treatment if it becomes necessary, does not constitute a positive choice.

While it can be hard for some of us to imagine why planned unassisted birth would seem like an attractive option, looking at the USA's maternal mortality rate (currently 28 deaths per 100,000, in comparison with the UK's eight and Sweden's four) it is clear that, although the mortality rate is still low compared with developing countries, there are reasons to be concerned about accessing care within a system where more women are dying – a near threefold increase in the past 25 years.

The reasons why so many American women are dying in childbirth are complex and not entirely understood. However, a healthcare system that makes those on low incomes unable or frightened to access care, or that prevents them from getting the kind of care they believe is safe and appropriate, is a significant factor. The 2009 Amnesty International report 'Deadly Delivery', which calls maternal health in the US a 'human rights failure', agrees. It is worth noting that despite a bias in law, prosecution and medical practice towards the foetus, the US lags behind all 27 'wealthy' countries in its infant mortality rate, which is more than three times higher than that of Finland or Japan, even though there is significantly more healthcare spending in the US. Closer examination of the data shows that maternal and infant mortality rates have strong links to ethnic, social and economic status. In the US, African American women are four times more likely to die of pregnancy-related complications than white women. Amnesty reports that their babies also die far more often than their white counterparts.

Studies on rising maternal mortality[52] in the developed world have shown less significant, but nonetheless real, increases in a number of countries, though the latest audit suggests that in the UK the maternal mortality rate is on the decline again. Nevertheless, studies have pointed to a mix of factors contributing to an increasing number of mothers dying in the developed world, including older mothers, IVF, immigration, language barriers and rising caesarean section rates. Professor of Complex Obstetrics Susan Bewley suggests that a significant element in this is the increase in medical intervention. With one in three US women giving birth by caesarean section and nearly a quarter being induced, it may well be a factor in why women are dying there. Bewley asks in a recent essay, 'Is the pendulum swinging too far?' and suggests that 'harm may be caused in pursuit of absolute safety'.[54] It makes sense to me that at some point, perhaps a point we arrived at a while ago, current obstetric practice reached the limit of what can be achieved and genuine innovation will be needed to drive the mortality rates back down. Part of that innovation may be as simple as not intervening so routinely in pregnancy and birth.

It is easy to be complacent about financial barriers to reproductive health in the UK, but a look at those at the edges of society shows those barriers sadly exist here too. Octavia Wiseman, a midwife at a central London hospital, has worked with undocumented women living 'illegally' in the UK. Legislation now instructs NHS trusts to present a vulnerable woman, often at the lowest end of the socioeconomic scale, with a bill of between £1,100 and £4,000 for her maternity care.

Trusts are also advised to employ debt-collection agencies to recover unpaid costs. We can't underestimate the impact on women and babies, whose 'illegal' status already makes a more complex pregnancy and birth more likely. Wiseman describes answering the phone to one of her caseload women, who tearfully told her of the £1,300 bill she had received following a termination for rare and terrible foetal abnormalities.[55]

The impact of maternity charges on migrant women is finally beginning to get a small degree of recognition and a number of UK advocacy groups are coming together to highlight the issue. Doctors of the World (which runs a drop-in clinic attended by migrant pregnant women in London) released a report in 2015 on the experiences of migrant women receiving maternity care. They highlighted the fact that the general migrant population who attend their clinics are deterred from accessing antenatal care for fear of getting into debt or being arrested. The report also detailed the significant administrative barriers faced by migrants trying to seek care. They are frequently asked to produce documentation that they simply don't have, and there's often confusion from those trying to implement policy on how to actually apply it.

Doctors of the World say that they, 'found evidence that the pregnant migrant women who access the London drop-in clinic in the majority of cases did not have a GP, despite being in the UK for on average 4.6 years at the time of delivery.' In the majority of cases these women were delaying their antenatal care and having fewer than the recommended number of antenatal appointments. It's easy to see why this group is at increased risk of pregnancy-related complications. Indeed, two of the 35 women that Doctors of the World were able to follow up sadly lost their babies. In both cases they received a bill for their hospital care.[56]

It's unacceptable that policy is forcing migrant women out

of maternity care and towards an uncertain and unsafe future. Sadly, the situation in the UK could be about to become worse, unless a new Department for Health proposal is successfully challenged – likely on human rights grounds. The proposal seeks to extend the current overseas visitors charging regime from secondary to primary and emergency care. This would mean that some vulnerable migrant women would face charges for using Accident and Emergency services and attending the GP, in addition to existing charges for seeing a midwife antenatally or postnatally and the costs of their care during childbirth.

Birthrights' response to the Department of Health consultation set out the key concerns. The existing charging rules are already misinterpreted and further charges could increase the likelihood of vulnerable women being denied care or being afraid to access it. Birthrights has already advised a number of pregnant women who have been mistakenly told that they cannot access care without payment in advance, and pregnant women with irregular immigration status already face difficulties registering with GPs. There is little doubt that the proposals would make all these things worse, increasing confusion for women and leading to reluctance to access services, not to mention poorer health outcomes.

Overseas visitors charging continues to be presented as a vital cost-saving measure, which tabloid stories on 'health tourism' seek to underline. In reality the significant expenditure related to implementing charging in primary care could mean that the costs to the taxpayer of this system greatly outweigh any financial benefits. Additional costs are almost certain to be incurred from delayed treatment, as women are likely to need more expensive intervention due to complications or a conservative approach to their unmonitored pregnancy. Add to this the cost of pursuing debts from people who may never be able to repay them, and the financial impact of defending possible legal challenges, and it's hard to accept that this proposal is designed to save money.

As Amnesty and Doctors of the World's work shows, fears about paying for care can lead to fewer women seeking care that they want and need. UK midwives have already documented what they term 'risky behaviour' (such as booking under someone else's name, or avoiding antenatal care entirely) on the part of undocumented women trying to access maternity care without incurring financial penalty. This behaviour can lead to uncertainty about blood type, HIV status, pregnancy history and more and makes it difficult (and eventually more expensive) to keep women and their babies safe.

In the UK, asylum-seeking and refugee women account for 14 per cent of maternal deaths despite comprising only 0.5 per cent of the population.[57] A 2013 report by Maternity Action and the Refugee Council looked at their experiences of pregnancy and birth and found that the UK Border Agency dispersed them repeatedly during their pregnancies, interrupting their care, depriving them of companions for birth and making it less likely they would have an interpreter or be able to build a relationship with a midwife. Rayah Feldman, author of the report, was struck by the indifference to healthcare within the asylum support system. Despite working daily on inequalities for women, she was 'shocked' by how they were treated during the dispersal process. She is clearly moved and motivated by how difficult it is for these women when they are arbitrarily shunted away from family, partners, other sources of practical and emotional support and their healthcare professionals.

Even when adequate healthcare provision is theoretically made, these limited examples shed light on how some women in these systems are still vulnerable. Safe, appropriate care that meets their needs simply does not exist.

Consent

Life-saving or not, the rising tide of intervention in birth has brought with it an uncomfortable truth. A woman's right to understand any proposed intervention, and then consent or decline, is being ignored on a regular basis around the world. Sometimes accidentally, sometimes deliberately.

Kimberley Turbin[58] has first-hand experience of obstetric violence.[59] Her case is unusual as her baby's birth was filmed and posted on YouTube. At the end of her labour Kimberley is immobilised by an epidural, her legs are in stirrups and her vagina is exposed. The doctor is gowned and masked, which is routine in US births but unnecessary and unheard of in the UK today outside of an operating theatre. She pushes for a while and then her doctor (Dr Alex Abbassi) says it's time for an episiotomy, a medical procedure that involves a surgical cut to Kimberley's perineum to speed up the birth.

She is upset and asks why, stating, 'We haven't even tried' and 'Don't cut me'. Her baby is not in distress and is beginning to emerge, but Abbassi's manner is aggressive. He doesn't give her clear answers and waves the episiotomy scissors around her vagina despite his knowledge that Kimberley is a two-time rape victim. As she resists, he becomes angry, shouting, 'Listen: I am the expert here!' On her next contraction, Kimberley's mother says, 'Don't worry, you just do it, Doctor.' The doctor performs an episiotomy without her consent. Instead of the usual inch-long cut, the scissors snip through her flesh again and again; 12 times in total. Her baby is born soon after.

Understandably, Kimberley is traumatised, as well as suffering pain and complications resulting from the cuts made in her perineum. Her initial letter of complaint resulted in no action and she has received no reply. She was initially unable to engage a lawyer to represent her in a lawsuit as the baby was unharmed. Legal precedent is not on her side, as in a 2003 negligence case in which an obstetrician performed an episiotomy without consent, the ruling went in the obstetrician's favour.[60]

However, thanks to the support of US advocacy organisations Improving Birth and Human Rights in Childbirth, a crowdfunding campaign has raised $14,000 to engage high-profile civil rights lawyer Mark Merin to represent her. In June 2015 Kimberley filed a complaint against Dr Abbassi for assault and battery. The case has potential to set an important precedent. 'This is an historic action,' says Mr Merin. 'Today, legal protections for American women in childbirth are uncertain—but with Ms Turbin's case, I intend to show that there are, indeed, real consequences when providers inflict harm on vulnerable patients.'[61]

Whether Kimberley's doctor's actions were medically mandated or not, they clearly constitute assault. Moreover, there appears to be no medical basis for the intervention. Kay Hardie, a UK independent midwife (whom I entrusted with my own care during my second pregnancy), explains that 'the only indication' for episiotomy with consent (outside of a birth that needs forceps or ventouse assistance) is significant concern about the baby's wellbeing. She adds, 'The foetal heart rate here is absolutely fine. Kimberley is told blatant lies about whether it is possible for her baby to be born without an episiotomy.' In fact, evidence and guidelines are now diametrically opposite to everything Kimberley was told, with episiotomies shown to *increase* not decrease the risks of serious tearing.

Kay's explanation for why Kimberley received 12 cuts instead of the usual single one is hard to hear. She says she has no doubts that the doctor 'was taking his revenge on her' for her attempts to refuse intervention, and points out that Kimberley should have been given a local anaesthetic before her episiotomy. Despite the epidural, she would have felt every cut. She describes this as 'appalling, shocking and bullying behaviour'. Article 5 of the Universal Declaration of Human Rights springs to mind: 'No one shall be subjected to torture or to cruel, inhuman or degrading treatment or punishment.'

After being stalled for a while (as Dr Abbassi has handed in his medical licence to the state and is no longer practising, claiming 'cognitive impairment'), in June 2016 LA County Superior Court Judge Benny C. Osorio ruled that Turbin v Abbassi could go ahead. As US-based Cristen Pascucci, founder of Birth Monopoly and vice-president of Improving Birth, explains, 'the judge was not interested in the other side's insinuations that the episiotomy was necessary and a decision for the doctor to make and ruled that the case was proper filed as a battery case not a negligence case'. The judge inquired why there were so many people in the courtroom, and Improving Birth President Dawn Thompson promptly informed his clerk that this is an unprecedented case of national interest about the legal rights of childbearing people, and that the women in the courtroom represented a cross-section of Kimberly's supporters. Asked how she feels, Kimberly said, 'I feel like crying. That the judge agreed it was a battery makes me feel validated.'

Kimberly is raising money for her ongoing legal case and has only raised 30 per cent of her crowdrise.com target so far. The Improving Birth team are encouraging donations with a shocking statistic, 'if every American woman who had a non-consented episiotomy in the year 2013 alone gave just 50 cents, Kimberley could easily fund the entire cost of the case – estimated at between \$50,000 and \$100,000 so far'.

I find it hard to understand why there hasn't been more coverage of Kimberley's story and wonder how much that has to do with an unwillingness to engage with childbirth as a women's rights issue. Elisa Albert seems to agree, believing that while rape is no longer culturally acceptable 'obstetric violence is the last culturally acceptable form of violence against women'. As Cristen Pascucci almost pleads, 'whether or not you have or want children please don't ignore the reality it is still permissible, in 21st-century America, to tell a grown woman to shut up, lie back, and not question what's done to her body.'[62]

I hope that this case will soon make legal protections for American women in childbirth far more concrete, as although Kimberley's case is extreme, some of her experiences are far from isolated. The 2006 Listening to Mothers Survey of US women reported that a staggering 73 per cent of mothers who received an episiotomy felt they hadn't consented to it. The survey hasn't been replicated in the UK, but the 2013 survey by Birthrights demonstrated that, seemingly to a lesser degree, consent issues are also a reality for UK women. Some 24 per cent of those who had an instrumental birth said they had not consented to the procedure.

It was not until after her second baby was born that Londoner Anne (well-informed, down-to-earth, with a successful career) was able to describe to me how deeply her first child's birth had affected her and the mother-baby relationship. Anne didn't feel she ever gave fully informed consent to an episiotomy, forceps and stitches which, in retrospect, were perhaps unnecessary.

No one was really treating me like a human being who might have feelings about what was going on. It didn't feel like anyone was trying to help me. It felt like I was in a process that was bigger than me, and I just had to go along with it without making too much fuss. It's not that they were malevolent towards me; it was just that they didn't care about me at all, except as a vessel for the baby.

After some tries at pushing, two obstetricians wandered in and said, 'At this stage we'd recommend forceps'. I assumed the baby must be in trouble. I felt they were the experts, I should go along with it; it would be selfish of me to go against their expertise and possibly harm my baby. Afterwards, going through my notes with the head of midwifery, I discovered the baby was fine throughout.

It sounds stupid, but I didn't realise that I would have to have an episiotomy. I think they mentioned 'we will have to do a cut', or something, but I didn't realise what a big deal an episiotomy was. Only when the midwives came for the home visits and checked my stitches did I properly realise I had stitches. It went on to be excruciatingly painful; so painful I would nearly faint or be sick. I never looked at it. I couldn't look at it for at least six months. It made me feel physically sick to think of it, let alone look at it.

After baby L was born, Anne couldn't face her family.

It seemed like such an enormous, unspeakable thing had happened to me. I didn't know where to begin. I didn't feel like I could talk about it at all and I wouldn't let my parents visit. I felt that I couldn't share their happiness and I had a responsibility to keep it together because I was a mother to a baby now. Really, I felt like I'd walked through the Valley of the Shadow of Death, and no one had any idea.

Anne's childbirth affected her well beyond those first days. 'I fell down a well of sadness and remained freaked out for about a year afterwards,' she explains, adding, 'I was alienated from the baby and completely daunted as a mother.' Anne's story is perhaps all the more upsetting knowing that she had so many advantages over so many other women in the UK system and yet this was still the result.

It is not only mothers who highlight these issues; healthcare workers know the problem all too well. Daniella, an NHS midwife taking part in research, explained that, for the most part, practices around seeking consent in the UK had improved, but that she had 'seen the other extreme where there's been absolutely no mention of what's going to happen and women's bodies have been touched without any consent whatsoever'. In two cases she has seen women being held down to have interventions performed on them.

In March 2015 the UK's Supreme Court powerfully affirmed women's right to autonomy in childbirth in the case of Montgomery v Lanarkshire Health Board. Allowing the appeal from the Scottish courts by a woman whose baby suffered shoulder dystocia in labour, the Supreme Court held that women have a right to information about 'any material risk' in order to make autonomous decisions about how to give birth.

The judgement significantly clarified and expanded on what the courts believe constitutes consent. In this case the doctor did not mention the chance of shoulder dystocia (an emergency condition in which the baby's shoulders get stuck after the head is born) to Mrs Montgomery. This was despite the fact that she was a diabetic woman with an elevated risk of experiencing shoulder dystocia during childbirth. The doctor's rationale was that the risk of serious injury to the baby was very small and that if she did outline it, and the more significant risks to the mother, 'then everyone would ask for a caesarean section'.

In her judgement Baroness Brenda Hale said:

> In this day and age, we are not only concerned about risks to the baby. We are equally, if not more, concerned about risks to the mother. And those include the risks associated

with giving birth, as well as any after-effects. One of the problems in this case was that for too long the focus was on the risks to the baby, without also taking into account what the mother might face in the process of giving birth.[63]

Lady Hale continued, 'gone are the days when it was thought that, on becoming pregnant, a woman lost, not only her capacity, but also her right to act as a genuinely autonomous human being.'

The judgement made it clear that in order for a patient to make an informed decision, there must be a conversation between clinician and patient. This must be an in-person discussion, not via a leaflet, and must be a two-way conversation, not the delivery of a one-way opinion from clinician to patient. Furthermore, the midwife or doctor must explain the 'material risk' to the woman. A material risk is one to which a reasonable patient would attach significance. Material risk will differ from woman to woman and pregnancy to pregnancy, so her caregiver must get to know the woman's individual circumstances and take these in to account when counselling her.

Critically, the court emphasised that consent forms alone cannot constitute consent. It can only be granted if the woman can understand the information that's been imparted on her own terms.

While there has been concern that the Montgomery judgement could lead to more litigation, Elizabeth Prochaska believes that, 'far from threatening doctors with more claims, proper disclosure of risks should protect the medical profession from litigation and lead to patients bearing responsibility for their own decisions. Respect for patient autonomy means that patients take responsibility.' It could also provide a prompt to improve continuity of care, as the conditions for consent as set out in this judgement may be difficult for many clinicians to meet in the current overstretched and fragmented system. This case has the potential to positively transform ideas around consent, autonomy and the clinician/patient relationship in the UK.

The rhetoric of choice and reality of coercion

I had a very good pregnancy and my labour happened one beautiful October morning. The doctor didn't believe me when I said I think I might be having contractions, because I looked too smiley and laid-back. But when he did a vaginal examination, I was five centimetres open.

I asked if I could communicate my birthing wish list with him, and he wasn't happy with my act and said that he treats all women equally as if they were his own wife. That a piece of paper would not make a difference in his treatment for me. I was just admitted and, from then on, I was a patient with a very strict protocol and I was no different.

I had a quarrel with my doctor when I rejected the augmentation. They didn't even ask me if I wanted it because during admittance you sign a piece of paper where you agree with your doctor's choices, all of them, upfront. It was psychologically exhausting to argue in such a fragile state. I felt inferior and completely out of my comfort zone. The doctor even tried tricking me into an induction by using another word. After our second argument he decided to fulfil my wish.

I was admitted, changed clothes, had the enema, and I shaved earlier at home because I'd heard nurses scolding women for coming in 'all hairy'. After my no-induction wish was fulfilled I pretty much compromised on everything else. I had my water mechanically broken; I had an episiotomy.

The labour was lasting more than three pushes,

everybody got frantic. The midwife told me the baby will suffocate, the doctor yelled, 'Come on, this is no joke any more!' and laid down all his weight on my stomach. Thinking of it in retrospect, I didn't have adequate informing on what to do; the doctor just said that I will know when the time comes to push. I had skin-to-skin contact immediately after birth for a quick second. I saw her again after four hours.

I have much greater insight with all of this experience and I am really hoping my next birth to go more natural. Also, I will continue arguing and this time I don't plan on sparing my strength too much. After all, we women have strength for all things necessary.

Amira is a first-time mother who recently gave birth in Sarajevo. While she doesn't draw out specific incidents of intervention against her will or without her consent, it's easy to see from her story how the rigid system she entered prevented her from giving birth the way she wanted, despite many of her requests being standard fare in other countries. A UK student midwife, who didn't wish to be named, explained the more subtle pressure felt by many women to do what they are told in labour: 'Women are made to feel so terrible if they don't conform and they're talked about within the staff room, you know, "I can't believe she hasn't done that" or "I can't believe she has done this". If you don't conform you are stereotyped into being a "bad woman".'[64]

As well as the maternity system imposing an expectation that women will conform and adopt the role of a compliant 'good girl' (a phrase that is often used in an attempt to soothe and encourage labouring women), it also exposes women to the reality of coercion. Being a 'good girl' is the opposite of being a 'bad mother'.

Ruth-Anna Macqueen (a mid-level obstetric doctor) believes UK obstetrics has moved forwards dramatically from its 'patriarchal history', and describes the profession now and 30 years ago as 'worlds apart'. She explains that in the UK, 'the majority of doctors currently training in obstetrics are female and many of us have had children and/or experienced miscarriage, stillbirth, neonatal deaths or traumatic birth ourselves'. She thinks this has led to many positive changes in the profession and that, across medicine in general, the concept of informed choice as opposed to paternalism is firmly embedded and included extensively in training.

However, Polly, an NHS consultant midwife, describes the clash between what is presented to women and what they receive, explaining that 'often you see the word "offer" – induction was "offered", something was "offered" – but it's not offered really'. Polly points to how the word 'offer' suggests something you can easily accept or decline, when that is often far from the case.

Studies have found that our supposed focus in the UK on 'woman-centred care' (something that appears repeatedly in policy documents) 'provides something in between a guarantee and an illusion of control for women becoming mothers for the first time'. Despite an official shift towards women's right to choose their pattern of maternity care, 'there was little evidence of women in the second [more recent] study being able to make meaningful informed choices'.[65]

Policy, law, rhetoric and training are reinforcing the importance of choice. Progress is being made, but the system in which this sits still exposes women daily to a lack of meaningful choice. Placed under extraordinary pressure to get mothering and the start to it 'right', women understandably buy into the rhetoric and attach further significance to the choices they wish to make around childbirth. For some, issues of self-worth are intertwined with the dignity they are afforded and the autonomy they can express during the process. A discovery, through bitter experience, that the maternity system they enter is structured in a way that often restricts choice, and can be toxic to women, is potentially harmful. That it then actively prevents many women from experiencing the kind of 'normal' birth that they will have been told repeatedly while pregnant is best for them and their babies can add such a mismatch between expectation and reality that it becomes almost intolerable.

Place of birth: home

Choice of place of birth has become one of the most politicised, over-discussed and sometimes distracting issues in maternity care. The physical nature of the choice in question, and the implicit values the chooser is ascribed upon making it, mean that it is difficult to discuss reasonably and impartially. As I'll go on to discuss in chapter 6, choosing a place of birth has become bound up in ideological birth talk that belies the fundamental rights that underpin it.

In February 2016 a National Review of Maternity Services in England published its report with a focus on community-based services, teamwork and 'personalised' care. The £3,000 personal maternity budget (a very small segment of the pilot proposals) was immediately pounced on by the press. 'Mothers-to-be will be handed £3000 by the NHS to buy the services of private midwives under plans to cut the number of hospital births' said *The Times*[66]. 'Why NO first-time mother should have a home birth' reported *The Daily Mail*.[67] Only two weeks later, on 15 March, *The Daily Mail* provided an example of how judgement abounds around all birth choices, describing one of the reasons for a rise in caesarean section rates as 'requests from women who are "too posh to push"'.[68]

As I set out in chapter 3, women's right to choose where they give birth is protected under Article 8 – the right to private life. This is a qualified right, which means it can only be limited if there are legitimate and proportionate reasons for doing so. If an NHS trust refuses to provide a homebirth service, for example, or has not set up adequate contingency plans to avoid staffing shortages in busy periods, this could be a breach of Article 8. A key aspiration of the National Maternity Review is that all women should have access to a choice of where they give birth by 2020. Yet all women should already reasonably expect this choice, based on Department of Health policy that came into effect in 2009 and the Human Rights Act.[69]

The uncomfortable reality is that some trusts in England are currently failing to provide any homebirth service or refusing to staff one adequately. At Kings Lynn hospital in Norfolk, the homebirth service has been suspended since 2013, citing staffing issues and low uptake among women. As the local trust also has no midwife-led unit, women who want to minimise routine intervention are left to choose between travelling long distances in labour, birthing unassisted, employing independent midwives at significant personal cost or attending the obstetric-led unit where almost half of low-risk women experience intervention in birth. The hospital has been reported to its regulator and legal action is being considered, with one woman receiving compensation following a complaint to the Ombudsman after having to pay an independent midwife to ensure she could have a homebirth.

In Cambridge the situation is less clear and reflects the position in many parts of the country, as local doula Maddie McMahon explains. After a period of uncertainty about whether the local hospital would provide a homebirth service at all (due to a lack of sufficient staff), a lone community midwife is now on call for homebirths, though during her shift she is working on the midwife-led unit.

Though some women are now encouraged to book a homebirth, others are positively discouraged by their midwives and doctors. Guilt, that ever-present layer on top of women's choices, is being used in Cambridge to prevent some women from accessing a choice that is being heavily promoted by national policy and is supported by evidence. Some women are told that calling a midwife out from the hospital could leave other women in the hospital without care. As McMahon explains, 'the burden of guilt falls squarely on the homebirther, yet women planning hospital births aren't told they may be preventing a midwife attending a homebirth, or required to sit through a long speech detailing the risks of hospital birth.'

More frequently under this new system women are being told that if there are no staff available, or the unit is closed, they will have to give up their homebirth plans at the last minute. This attitude has an impact on the feeling about homebirth locally. Ten years ago the homebirth rate in Cambridge was reaching 6 per cent (small, but three times the national average). It now sits at under 1 per cent. Maddie McMahon asks, 'Do we blame women for not demanding homebirths, or point the finger at a system that appears to be discouraging it?' She finds it impossible to believe that the women of Cambridge are suddenly less enamoured of homebirth than those in other areas. When we have so much evidence that continuity of carer leads to massive rises in homebirth rates, McMahon's contention is that we should be working on making sure women are able to build close, trusting relationships with a named midwife or two during pregnancy and are encouraged to decide in labour where they would like to have their baby.

Yet homebirth still seems to inspire some of the most extreme and negative reactions to women's childbirth choices. When discussing recommendations that women should be enabled to choose out of (as well as in) hospital places of birth on national news, my measured response and positive attitude to homebirth for those that want it led to me being called a 'zealot'. Homebirth is a particularly unacceptable choice in the current climate around birth and negative discussions are often bound up in presumptions around the demographic of women who access homebirth.

As McMahon adds:

> There is a perception that access to homebirth is a problem of the privileged. Yet this is far from the truth. Homebirth – or more precisely out-of-hospital birth – is a vital issue in the realm of women's rights. Victims of abuse, rape and birth trauma often feel psychologically much safer away from environments where the power dynamic can be challenging for them. Women suffering grief, bereavement or mental health issues may all feel safer away from hospital. Practical concerns such as childcare or lack of social support may make homebirth more attractive and a background that has taught a woman to distrust the 'authorities' may mean she benefits from supportive care in her own environment.

If women with more education and from more privileged socio-economic groups are accessing homebirth, we have to wonder whether the patchy provision, lack of local support and constant service suspensions are partly to blame for this skewed uptake.

Unassisted birth and social services

> When I had my first baby I knew nothing about birth. I was lucky though and found myself pushing my daughter out in the birth pool before the midwife returned – just

six hours after arriving at hospital. When I found out I was expecting my second it felt completely natural and normal to have minimal medical involvement. I felt very early on that I wanted to birth unassisted. I declined routine scans but at every appointment I was met with pressure to have one.

I spoke to a Supervisor of Midwives and let her know about my plans to give birth unassisted and I wrote a letter confirming this. I thought they were being supportive, however a few weeks later, out of the blue, I received a letter from social services who had made an appointment to see me. My husband and I attempted to cancel the appointment but could not get in touch with anyone and so I wrote a long letter detailing the law and guidelines surrounding my choice to freebirth, whilst also declining their services.

Two weeks passed and I did not hear from them. In that time, my son was born unassisted at home in the bath. It was a short, intense labour and a birth experience which was grounding and profound. He was born at 12.30am, we were all in bed by 4am and I enjoyed this blissful time until the evening of the sixth day when I received a phone call from a social worker. What ensued was a nightmarish week of repeated visits from social services – sometimes accompanied by police officers.

Though we were told initially that this was nothing to do with our birth plans we found out that the referral had come directly from the midwives and was because we were planning an unassisted birth. Eventually the case against us was shown to be unfounded and was closed, but not before it had been escalated to a full-on child protection case concerning both of our children. It was terrifying. I was panicked and distressed by the visits and the persistence *needed from us to get the case closed was exhausting. It was very difficult to return to normal and I was so grateful for my exhilarating birth memories to return to.*

What I find so difficult is that birth is shrouded in a political climate but these are very personal choices. Sometimes people feel backed into birthing unassisted because of fear – but this wasn't me. I was making a positive decision and chose a valid birth option on the wide spectrum that should be available. I understand why people misinterpret freebirth and why this is difficult for some. In a culture where we have difficulty accepting homebirth as normal, freebirth must seem outlandish to the majority.

Melissa Thomas had her second baby in 2012. Her story is illustrative of the experiences some women and their families have faced during and after planned or accidental unassisted birth. Over the past three years Birthrights has seen a worrying rise in enquiries from families who have experienced social services involvement in legitimate decisions around unassisted birth or declining of routine intervention. In more than one case apologies have eventually been received by the families for the trauma caused by this involvement, although the tendency to use social services as a threat to coerce women into complying with policy does not seem to have abated.

Social services as a tool for coercion featured in a 2012 case concerning Southern General Hospital in Glasgow. The hospital was eventually forced to apologise to a woman who was bullied into taking precautionary antibiotics before birth. After a two-year fight she took her case to the Scottish Public Services Ombudsman and the hospital admitted that she had been threatened with social services action and having her baby removed from her care if she didn't consent to antibiotics that she didn't want or need. Such undue pressure effectively invalidated the consent she gave to the intervention and the Ombudsman upheld her complaint, stating that she 'did not properly consent to the treatment administered and was wrongly put under extraordinary pressure during labour when she was in a very vulnerable situation'.

In addition to prompting social services referrals, there's a lack of understanding around women's rights to decline care before, during or after birth. Though, as discussed earlier, unassisted birth can be a symptom of a system of maternity care that doesn't meet women's needs, for some it represents a valid and positive personal decision. As p.144 explains in more detail, no woman in England, Scotland or Wales can be compelled to accept any form of antenatal or in-labour care from midwives or doctors. Nevertheless, some medical professionals seem unaware of the law around freebirth and women are repeatedly told that declining medical care during pregnancy is against the law and will trigger referrals to the social services or even the police.

In February 2015 Melissa Thomas went on to have another baby without medical assistance. This time she was able to navigate the system with a supportive Supervisor of Midwives. 'For all its pain and how unbelievably mentally and physically challenging the birth was I knew it was exactly the experience I had needed. It gave me great personal insight and was a defining moment in my life. It brought together all of my birth experiences and seemed to reunite something within me,' explains Melissa.

She adds that if she were to offer any advice to other freebirthing women seeking support from their local NHS team she 'would recommend that they deal directly with their Supervisor of Midwives, that they utilise the support available from organisations such as Birthrights and the Association for the Improvement of Maternity Services in finding appropriate ways to maintain friendly open relationships, whilst having firm boundaries and clarity about what they want and expect from their care.'

If any challenges are faced, she suggests understanding the process of requesting a midwife capable of meeting your individual needs and escalating to supervisors and managers where needed. Melissa believes that planning a freebirth doesn't have to be a complex fight between a person's needs and the system.

Elective caesarean section

The challenges women face when trying to choose where and how to give birth are often presented most urgently in relation to out-of-hospital birth. However women at the other end of the spectrum of birth choice face very similar access issues and comparable levels of judgement. Far from being on opposite sides of a supposed birth divide, homebirthing women and those choosing a caesarean section have much to unite them.

Choosing a caesarean section for non-medical reasons can bring women into a complex wrangle between physical and mental health, maternity policy and health professionals' personal biases and preferences. Page 148 of this book outlines in detail how women's rights impact on requests for a caesarean section. In brief and simplistic terms, women do not have a specific right to a caesarean, but bearing in mind the human rights expectations all women should enjoy, such a request should be considered carefully and individually for each woman and the physical risk of the procedure and elevated costs compared to a vaginal birth should be balanced against the woman's wishes and mental health.

The NICE guidelines give a best-practice outline that suggests women are referred for counselling if they request a caesarean for non-medical reasons, but that their request should ultimately be granted. Obstetricians can refuse to perform the procedure, but they should refer to a colleague to fulfil the woman's request.

Sadly, many women find the pathway to a birth they believe will fit their personal circumstances far less smooth. Some complain that the counselling is unwanted or coercive; others that the process of requesting a caesarean is traumatic and drawn out. Increasingly, hospitals tell women they have a 'no maternal request caesarean policy', which is hard to justify (like all applications of blanket policies). Women speak of judgement and confusion from the midwives and doctors they meet, of deliberate obstruction to their wishes and a routine dismissal of their fears and concerns.

When 29-year-old Lauren O'Malley-Dean had her first baby in September 2015, she wanted to give birth by caesarean section. Though there was no physical reason for her choice, her family's birth history and her previous mental health problems were at the forefront of her mind. Aware that she was at higher risk of postnatal depression, she was concerned that a traumatic birth could trigger a depressive episode. 'The first person I had to convince was my midwife,' Lauren explains. 'I went to my booking appointment armed with my reasons, but was told I'd most likely have an ordinary birth so not to worry. So I asked to speak to a consultant.'

Lauren was told by the junior doctor she later saw that it was best to wait and see. Then the consultant 'told me I was being silly, which made me feel like a child, despite repeatedly telling him my mental health was a priority. If my husband hadn't been there fighting my corner I would probably have caved and agreed to a natural birth.' Lauren had to justify and insist on her choice twice more, including on the morning of the birth itself. Despite the difficulties she faced, she now believes an elective caesarean was totally the right choice for her.

Danielle had her second baby in 2015 and faced similar struggles to Lauren. After a previous vaginal birth that left her with serious physical and mental trauma, she knew she could not give birth vaginally again.

> I put forward my choice to give birth by caesarean at my first antenatal appointment. I didn't even question whether or not I was 'entitled' to a caesarean, I naively thought that I would be allowed the birth of my choice. In fact, I assumed it would be recommended for me.
>
> At the appointment I was told I'd 'never get' a caesarean. I felt shocked, angry and scared. Could I really be forced into a vaginal delivery? The midwife had been blasé, telling me 'second babies are much easier'. When I told her my son had almost died after delivery, she said he was 'unlucky'. When I told her I was left with bladder and bowel prolapses at the age of 23 she didn't seem to care.
>
> I knew that I was not going to be made to do this. I got informed, read some books and visited the Birthrights website. I never, ever lost that feeling of 'this is right for me'. I just knew it in my gut. Once I had armed myself with a copy of the 'Maternal Request Caesarean Section' part of the NICE guidelines, and written a letter outlining why I wanted the procedure, I went back to the midwife.
>
> She took me a bit more seriously though I could tell she deeply disapproved of my choice. I wanted all those things we are told are bad: the noisy machines, the bright lights, the room full of people, the drugs, the instruments... I wanted it all, I needed it to feel safe. To make sure my baby was safe. I will say here that I felt very angry with her.
>
> She eventually agreed to refer me to the consultant who, to my surprise, told me she completely understood

why I was choosing a caesarean and began pulling consent papers out of her desk for me to sign. But when I did see the midwife again and asked her to ring to book my caesarean date she said it was too early. She continued to put me off until I reached 37 weeks. A few days later I got a letter through the door saying my section had been booked for 40+2 – over a week beyond my specified gestation of 39 weeks. This was not acceptable to me as it was clear that there was a good chance I could go into labour before this date resulting in an emergency procedure or having an unwanted vaginal delivery – both of which would increase risk to myself and my baby.

I was 38 weeks by this point and extremely upset, I felt I had no choice but to play a waiting game and the reassuring risk/benefit ratios I had been using to prop up my decision were slipping away the closer I got to my due date. I had nightmares about going into labour.

I got in touch with PALS (the Patient Advisory and Liaison Service) and the next day they rang to say they had sorted it out. At 39 weeks exactly my daughter was born by caesarean in perfect condition. The day itself went very smoothly. I was nervous but it was nothing compared to the debilitating fear I felt when I thought about having to have a vaginal birth. My daughter was well, I was well, and it was only after I had that joyous birth experience that I realised how much the trauma of that first birth had affected me. It had damaged my bond with my son and ruined my self-esteem.

Ultimately my story had a happy ending. But throughout my pregnancy I was powerless about choices that I instinctively felt were my right to make. I kept thinking, if women are allowed to choose to have an abortion, why am I not able to choose how I give birth? In the Victorian era

*women were thought to be ruled by their wombs. It seems
to me that, when it comes to birth, we still are.*

Too fat, too old, too everything: birth centres

Birth centres (be they freestanding midwifery-led units or
alongside units within existing maternity centres) are often
presented to women as the 'best of both worlds'. A middle
ground where women who want to be in a medical setting,
but are keen to give birth without intervention, can feel safe
and have their wishes respected.

In the UK they are usually beautifully appointed with double
beds, dimmable lights, music, a birth pool, a range of bean bags,
birth stools, ropes and other tools for active birth. Birth centres
often have relaxed policies about visitors and allow partners to
stay overnight after the baby is born. They are often in stark
contrast to the small and basic 'delivery rooms' of the labour
ward with their many rules and conventions – where nine out
of ten women in England actually end up giving birth.

In a 2013 Royal College of Midwives report on
'freestanding midwife-led units in England and Wales' the
authors found there were 59 freestanding midwife-led units
(FMUs) compared with 53 in April 2001. The rising number
belies a constant uncertainty in service provision, as during
these twelve years 30 new units opened, but 21 others were
permanently closed.

The number of women birthing in these settings remains
small. In England around 12,000 women have their baby in
an FMU, less than 2 per cent of women giving birth in an
English NHS setting. In England the majority of FMUs have
200–300 births a year, whereas in Wales they have fewer
than 50 births a year.

Midwife-led units are being promoted by policy and
guidance at all levels. This is unsurprising given the

comparatively low rates of intervention, high levels of satisfaction and excellent outcomes for mother and baby. However, with such a small uptake many freestanding units face closure and there seems to be near-constant (and no doubt justified) anxiety among the midwives that run and work in these units that unless they 'get their numbers up' their places of work will be shut down. The difficulty in increasing the number of women is often presented as being indicative of a lack of interest from women or concerns about safety locally. These factors may play a role, though to my mind they are complicated by a 'chicken or egg' argument and are often caught up local maternity power struggles.

I would argue that the real barriers to raising the numbers of women giving birth in midwife-led units stem from the litigation culture around maternity services, the fear it produces and the increasingly popular view of the mother as a risky, flawed vessel at odds with her baby. In this context there are very few women deemed 'low-risk enough' to birth in these units by the time they go into labour. This was Karen Birch's experience when she had her first baby in January 2016.

I really wanted to go to the local birth centre. My best friend had both her babies there and it has such a good reputation. I'm frightened of hospitals and needles so I didn't want to be on the labour ward, but I was also scared of the pain of childbirth so I wanted a birth pool, gas and air, pethidine if I needed and really good support from the midwives. It looked so much nicer than the labour ward too. Newer and with better facilities. It just seemed like the obvious choice.

I felt I was being put off and placated every time I tried to talk about where I wanted to give birth. Eventually at 34 weeks I was made an appointment to see if I fitted the 'criteria' for the birth centre. I went along and was told in no uncertain terms that I didn't. I was too fat (by one BMI point) and too old (by two weeks). At the time I didn't know how to challenge it. I just felt awful and totally terrified.

I did think about a homebirth quite seriously then but I'm quite far away from the hospital and it didn't feel safe for me. Neither did being on the labour ward but for different reasons. I felt I was being forced between a rock and a hard place. To choose between being physically safe and feeling ok mentally. It was so unfair that the middle ground just wasn't open to me. And there are so many more mothers who are older or overweight these days so why weren't we being catered for?

I decided to go to hospital in the end. I was induced and had a failed ventouse, forceps and eventually a crash caesarean section after days of labour. I think I was too scared to go into labour by myself and go to this place I hadn't chosen. I was right to be scared. I have flashbacks and disturbed sleep now and am seeking treatment. I'll never have another baby.

Karen's story of not fitting the criteria is one I hear all the time. One midwife in Kent, who didn't want to be named, told me:

...the criteria for the midwife-led unit is getting narrower and narrower. It's because the hospital is frightened of legal action if they let the wrong woman in but I'm beginning to wonder if it's also a way of shutting these units down by stealth. I do wonder why the lawyers aren't worried about a woman suing us because she felt forced to give birth at home to have her needs met and then suffers a bad outcome.

Whether women want to birth alone, at home, in a birth centre or choose an elective caesarean – their decisions are often at the very bottom of a hierarchy of policy, power, control and risk-management. Somehow a range of these external forces on childbirth have combined to make it difficult for women who want to avoid unnecessary intervention to do so. With a focus on reducing the rising caesarean section rate (which is at least in part the fault of infrastructure, practice and culture), women who want to access caesareans for non-medical reasons become the easiest group to control. Instead of optimising the chances of women who want a vaginal birth, and making a planned caesarean possible for the small group of women who request it on non-medical grounds, all are being punished for the system's faults, whatever they choose. An unwanted and unnecessary emergency caesarean or forceps birth for the woman denied a homebirth or access to a birth centre. A stress-filled fight to get a caesarean agreed to for a woman who actually wants one.

It can be as difficult to access birth options at both ends of the spectrum and a heavy mental toll is levied on women who must relentlessly argue their case or accept something that doesn't feel safe to them. Women talk about safety and control with remarkable similarity whatever decision they are attempting to make. Yet conversations about these choices are often presented in an oppositional, confrontational and judgmental way, as if the groups have nothing in common. So why have women been distracted by arguing among themselves and consistently struggled to find unified ground on which to stand and defend their rights?

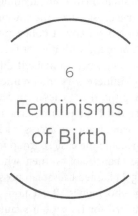

6

Feminisms
of Birth

Political and moral acts

If women find themselves under an unequal microscope when making life choices, this intensifies exponentially when they step into the realm of the reproductive. Dr Ellie Lee feels that one of the difficulties woman face in motherhood and childbirth is having every choice interpreted as a political or moral act.

Birth may be a significant part of the feminist jigsaw puzzle, but the pieces haven't yet slotted together in a comfortable way, despite huge advancements in women's rights over the past 100 years. I will go on to talk about worrying incursions into these, but the majority of women in the UK are now able to access contraception and the NHS will fund most abortions. Support for abortion among the general public is high, with a poll[70] showing around 80 per cent of us believe in legal abortion in all or most cases. The US is much more undecided. In a 2015 survey they were split almost equally into the pro-choice/anti-abortion camps, with 50 per cent describing themselves as pro-choice and 44 per cent as pro-life.[71]

Women have historically owned childbirth out of necessity and design. In the UK, it is only in the last 300 years that men have become prominent figures in the birth room and only in the last 100 that their presence has been widespread. Birth has been 'women's business' and our domain throughout history. Yet, despite women having claimed and owned the birth room until very recently, awareness of birth as a reproductive rights issue among women has been comparatively slow to emerge. Reproductive rights campaigning has, more effectively and more concentratedly, focused its gaze on abortion, contraception and sexual rights, with birth rights remaining the poor relation.

If we return to Lynn Paltrow's comment that it is pregnancy that provides the very excuse for the broad inequalities women face, it is unsurprising that it has been challenging to reconcile the wider feminist project with childbirth rights. Simultaneously, those who have advocated for women in a pregnancy and birth context have not always defined themselves as feminists. Sociologist Ann Oakley's writings on feminism and birth in the late 1970s and 80s highlighted the patriarchal nature of contemporary maternity care. She detailed a 'doctor knows best' paternalism that was all-pervasive, which wrestled from women the control of their bodies and the child-bearing process. Oakley's work followed grassroots movements such as the founding of the Society for the Prevention of Cruelty to Pregnant Women (now the Association for Improvements in the Maternity Services, AIMS) in 1960 and the Natural Childbirth Trust (now National Childbirth Trust) just before.[72]

Since then, historians like Tania McIntosh have suggested that this is too simple, acknowledging the often unseen 'private acts of feminism and power' in birth rooms across time and place. Martha Ballard, a midwife in rural Maine, kept a diary of her life and work between 1785 and 1812.

Her quiet but secure status, her bravery as she crossed raging rivers in storms to ensure Mrs Hewins was 'safe delivd of a Daughter',[73] her life as a businesswoman in her own right and the midwifery skills she possessed and taught are woven through her diary. A tiny slice of life exemplifying some of these private acts of feminism. Ballard's diary could easily serve as a document demonstrating the power of women in birth before a paternalistic system took it from them. It could just as easily be viewed as a record of the hardships and restriction of women before safety in birth was achieved and they were liberated from its pain and suffering. The same narratives can provide evidence for a range of often oppositional ways of looking at birth and the feminist issues it raises. A global, social history of birth and maternity care would take years to write in a sufficiently nuanced way. Instead, we tend to view these birth stories through our own political prisms.

The oppositional trend can perhaps be partly explained by the fact that women's lives and individual choices are instantly politicised and moralised in a way that men's aren't. Reproductive decisions can become highly controversial, as chapter 1 explained. 'Women who have abortions aren't trying to make a political statement,' says Dr Lee, and her comment could equally read: 'Women who have elective caesareans, epidurals, homebirths, unassisted births, bottle-feed or breastfeed their children until the age of four aren't trying to make political statements.' Nevertheless, we have become used to thinking this way. Women who express one opinion are accused of making another group feel guilty because, even if it isn't present (and oftentimes it is), a value judgement is instantly associated with a particular choice. One of the ways feminism has struggled to tackle the inequalities in birth is the overbearing presence of the political and moral lens in the argument.

My birth is not a feminist statement

In 2011 the 'Isis the Scientist' blog ran an article entitled 'Your home birth is not a feminist statement'.[74] Her title is compelling and important. Birth choices are not political statements. I've yet to find a woman making such an important choice just to make a point. What does seem to exist is the appropriation of birth choices to make a political statement, some of which are couched in the language of feminism. Childbirth educator Andrea Robertson, in an article with the heading 'The pain of labour – a feminist issue', describes the choice to have pain relief in labour in such a way:

> *Since this [pain in labour] is such a common experience it could be seen as comforting, a bond among women, a fundamental truth that confirms our special biological role and affirms the importance of our contribution to society. More often, however, it is seen as a blight, an unnecessary imposition, an affliction we must bear as the price for bearing children. This view, bolstered by the perception that pain is a symptom of disease and illness, has enabled medical men to convince us that pain is dispensable during birth, and is of no value, an evil to be cured with modern treatments and technology.[75]*

Her piece is one of many aligning a 'natural' birth movement with feminist statements, perhaps a reaction to the experience of the paternalistic approach of medicalised birth, but one guaranteed to make women who choose pain relief feel angry and alienated. This politicising of pain in labour illustrates the dangers of putting value judgements on birth choice. It also highlights the unintended outcomes of campaigning around a particular type of birth for all women, rather than individualised care for all.

The idea of pain as a positive statement about being a woman makes more sense in the context of the accidental consequences of early women's rights activists, and particularly those campaigning for the availability of an early pain relief method: Twilight Sleep. This involved injecting a mixture of scopolamine (a drug that causes amnesia) and morphine, and was promoted by the *Frauenkliniken* (women's clinic) in Germany from 1906 onwards. Touted as a miraculous drug providing painless childbirth, its use spread across the USA in the early 20th century. After US reporters wrote about '*Dämmerschlaf*' in a New York magazine (despite much controversy in the medical community), the demand for painless labour precipitated a campaign that saw the New England Twilight Sleep Association successfully petitioning hospitals to provide scopolamine for women locally.

In 1958, by which time Twilight Sleep had become standard fare in the US delivery room, the *Ladies' Home Journal* ran a short letter from an anonymous nurse entitled: 'Cruelty in the maternity wards'.[76] It sought investigation into 'the tortures that go on in the delivery room'. The series of readers' letters that followed pointed to the established practice of administering scopolamine routinely, without consent. Women often reacted to the drugs by entering a psychotic state, hallucinating and thrashing so wildly that they had to be tied to the beds. Wrists and ankles were left bleeding from restraints. Neighbours complained about the screams they were now privy to. Women found themselves subjected to routine episiotomies and forceps deliveries. They described partial, frightening recollections of their nightmarish treatment during birth and complete disconnection from their babies.

The reaction to this brutal treatment of women part-propelled one feminist figuring of childbirth, which sees the system as controlling, and promotion of 'natural' birth as a way to reclaim and empower. It goes some way to explain suspicion of pain relief among some feminist birth movements. That some of this movement reacts to an earlier campaign (by women) to liberate women from pain in labour is ironic and illustrates what happens when a prescriptive single-issue focus on a type of birth is privileged over care that allows women to honour their individual situations and wishes.

Understandably, many feminists have taken issue with the 'pain equals empowerment' idea. Returning to the 'Isis the Scientist' blog, while her title is easy to agree with she goes on to place a negative judgement on the choice of homebirth, making an anti-homebirth drive a political statement in itself. She adds:

> *Homebirth as a way to find a loving supportive environment and fight the enslavement of the patriarchy is absolute, utter nonsense. It's one of the only medical scenarios I can think of where women place health and welfare in jeopardy in order to feel 'in control' and avoid intervention.*

In the same way that Robertson confused the possible pros and cons of an individual choice with a political statement, Isis seems to believe that by choosing to birth at home a woman is attempting a feminist call to arms at personal cost. Moreover, like Robertson, she is critical of that choice. She finds it 'utter nonsense'.

The minutiae of blogs can seem like a distraction from the broader message here, but to me they illustrate the insidious and pervasive habit of confusing a woman's individual choice with broader issues. The faulty assumptions, clumsy use of feminism and presentation of motherhood and birth choices as constantly at war with one another, all play out in consulting rooms, media outlets and policy documents, once again distracting us from what is important when we look at women's rights in a reproductive context.

Those of us who believe that women shouldn't be discriminated against may disagree widely about how to prevent this. But surely we should be united under the banner of protecting autonomy and dignity? No type of birth is 'feminist'. By finding wider political action in such a personal health choice we undermine the very root of feminism. If we extrapolate Isis's logic, it seems she believes that all women should give birth in hospital and that those who don't are reckless. If we extrapolate Robertson's logic, it's easy to consider that those who give birth with pain relief have been brainwashed into making a choice that has deprived them of something essential to being a woman. Both are symptoms of a system that has always encouraged us to judge our choices along a political and moral spectrum. Sadly, some feminisms of birth have unwittingly become part of the problem they are trying to tackle.

The continuing stigmatisation of women's birth choices is inevitable, and I think those of us who are interested in reproductive rights need to make the case that women are best placed to make these intimate decisions. Whether it's pain relief, abortion, place of birth or consenting to intervention, once we have provided a care model that makes the broad range of choices possible and safe, society should leave it up to us and resist the urge to comment.

Individual v collective

So, is it possible to advocate for broader change without confusing the personal and the political and risk making women feel that their individual choices don't live up to pre-defined expectations?

Milli Hill, founder of the Positive Birth Movement (a network of nearly 300 groups across the world), believes it is. Hill says the movement tries 'not to focus on "natural" birth, but rather on what feels right for each individual woman', and sees its role as 'advocating for women's rights in childbirth and for women to get the births they really want, whatever that may be'.

Natalie Meddings, a UK-based doula, set up the website tellmeagoodbirthstory.com in 2000 with friend Kate Jones. After buddying one of her clients with a mother who had recently had a positive experience, Natalie saw the need for a way of reimagining the women's network. In our fractured communities where birth is most often viewed sensationally on television, rather than first hand in the community, Tell Me a Good Birth Story has over 800 women on its database ready to buddy anyone who feels they need support.

The service is intended partly to offer an antidote to an ideological view of birth. Natalie points to media messaging and some of the more misguided aspects of natural birth ideology as encouraging women to 'see childbirth like a kind of test'. Believing that birth should never be 'a competition with themselves or anyone else', she feels that certain 'types' of birth have become synonymous with a positive experience and sees 'a lot of pressure in the form of women preparing for birth like a job'.

Pauline Hull, co-author of *Choosing Cesarean*, also notes pressure being exerted on women who feel that 'births at home and in midwifery-led birth centres are not risk-free (no birth is), and yet they are more readily supported in the UK than caesarean at maternal request. Why? Because ideology is being allowed to trump evidence.'

Although there are debates around this evidence, it is easy to see how rhetoric around the idea of promoting a specific way of giving birth has grown up. With rising rates of unnecessary, emergency intervention, and increasing evidence that the pendulum has swung too far, there is a growing focus on how

111

to stem a tide of intervention, lower the caesarean rate and increase rates of vaginal and more specifically 'normal' or (as I prefer) physiological birth.

The UK's Royal College of Midwives (RCM) used to have a 'Campaign for Normal Birth', but recently and sensibly changed the title and focus of the campaign to the 'Better Births Initiative'. As Dr Rupa Chilvers explains, 'we took the decision in 2014 to expand the Campaign for Normal Birth to encompass the needs of all women being cared for in the maternity care system.' However, the new Better Births Initiative does continue to work on the theme of facilitating normal births and normality for all women as part of its remit. In addition, two more themes have been adopted, including increasing access to continuity of care and addressing health inequalities. The RCM's campaign sits among a decades-old tide of policy documents, as well as NHS England's 2014 vision for healthcare, all advocating birth options that maximise the chance of physiological birth.

Research supports these ambitions as matching what many women want, as well as improving safety for them. Yet changing the culture around birth without moralising individual choices is incredibly challenging. How can we say 'more women overall should be giving birth physiologically' without unwittingly pointing the finger at those who don't? At a societal level, a value judgement is placed on birth and reinforced with continuous messages that say physiological birth is best. We then enter a system that often makes physiological birth incredibly difficult for individuals to achieve, and all the while the choices they make are becoming part of the political yo-yo.

Brazil has become infamous for its human rights in childbirth failures and in spring 2014 the international media condemned the forced caesarean section of Adelir Carmen Lemos de Goes. The caesarean section rate in public hospitals is over 50 per cent. In the private sector it rises to well over 80 per cent. Fewer than 5 per cent of Brazilian women give birth without significant intervention, contrasting with 50 per cent of women in the UK. Valéria Fernandes, a Brazilian woman who planned a homebirth, sounds angry and bewildered when she talks about her experience of childbirth in 2013:

After my emergency caesarean section I felt broken and incompetent. I was sad for months; even now I cry when I remember. I would feel better if I was sure it was necessary, but I'm almost sure it was not. For that reason, my pain and frustration stay inside me. What I know is that my pain is mine and mine alone, most people would never empathise with me, because in my country c-section is the best way to be born and mothers are just receptacles, not persons with feelings. Or else, my only feelings should be, 'My baby is OK no matter what cost!'

She believes that most Brazilian women, encouraged by a for-profit, private obstetric lobby and the hardship that they may experience during vaginal birth in Brazil, see childbirth as a 'very painful moment; a very lonely one and one of great vulnerability'. Vaginal birth in particular is seen as being full of 'great suffering, danger and humiliation' and only 'for the poor or hippies'. In addition, Valéria feels women are encouraged to see caesareans as status symbols.

Women in public hospitals are often forced to give birth alone, their freedom of movement restricted and pain relief denied. The Birth in Brazil[77] study shows that, once again, those at the lowest end of the socioeconomic scale receive some of the worst care. In the private sector, where the overwhelming majority of women have caesarean sections, maternal satisfaction is higher, although this masks some unethical practices within it.

Despite this, I was surprised to discover that studies[78] show that most Brazilian women still want to avoid caesarean, citing the faster recovery time from vaginal birth. Trying to make positive vaginal birth a reality for Brazilian women is important not because of shiny ideologies, but because 73 per cent of Brazilian women don't want a caesarean. Yet achieving that without adding to the burden on the individual is hard.

Midwifery professor Hannah Dahlen thinks that it is possible to separate support for a woman's right to choose from promoting systemic change. As a practising midwife she believes 'you can't argue that you support choice in one aspect and not in another', and that 'it's exactly the same for homebirth, as it is for elective caesarean, as it is for abortion'. In Dahlen's eyes, a woman must be supported whatever she chooses and healthcare providers should have an obligation to ensure she is informed and understands the potential benefits and harms of what she is doing. Alongside that, there is what she alone understands about what risk means to her, and what the other non-clinical dangers and advantages are that might affect her decision. In Dahlen's experience, though, when women have access to truly individualised care provided inside social models, they most frequently want to pursue a physiological birth. Those who do not should be supported equally in their choice.

Among the women, healthcare providers and policymakers I have spoken to, one of the few ideas that brings almost universal consensus is the desperate need for more support across the child-bearing years. The evidence base, along with women's own demands, points to one-to-one midwifery care as answering that call for support. The increasing use of doulas and the evidence from a Cochrane Review on continuous support in labour are further telling markers of women's desire to be properly supported during a vulnerable time. Lindsey Middlemiss, Doula UK spokesperson, adds that 'much of our role is often being the person who understands that childbirth is a normal part of life, providing unspoken reassurance for expectant and labouring parents that all is well'. Perhaps because they bring back tools from our previous community lifestyles, Middlemiss believes one reason doulas are becoming popular is that 'experience and speech as means of sharing, which were traditionally the way female knowledge was passed on, have been largely sidelined in recent decades, but when it comes to learning about birth, nothing else works so well'.

Perhaps, as Dahlen suggests, it is this type of care that can unite different ideas about which is the 'right' way to give birth. If we put aside the one-track focus on intervention rates and 'normal' birth rates, and instead look at providing the right models of care and support choice, we will find women have safer, more fulfilling and less damaging experiences of birth, while maintaining the physical safety of mother and baby. This approach could link supposedly divergent feminist ideas around childbirth, and supersede policy and practitioner rhetoric that has pursued 'normal' birth as the desired outcome inside a system that effectively prevents it for many.

Humanity is the key to breaking down acceptance of practices that not only humiliate, imprison, endanger and abuse women, but eat away at their basic rights. In South America the extent of the problem has provoked a revolutionary solution and one that isn't bound up with too much ideology. The innovative humanising birth movement (resulting in government-sponsored programmes like the Stork Network in Brazil), and the many inspiring activists behind it, pushes for safe and quality care with a woman-centred, respectful approach at all times. Rather than privileging specific targets and outcomes, thus increasing pressure on the individual, the humanising birth movement aims to put basic human dignity back into childbirth. The impact and potential to shift the power balance means it is an approach now being watched and emulated around the world.

Senior midwife Nagela Santos of the Hospital Sofia Feldman in Belo Horizonte, Brazil, believes change is happening – at least in the public sector. Through the work of the humanising birth movement systemic change has led to a service that values the experiences of women within it and, as a byproduct, the caesarean section rate is lower than in many London hospitals (26.6%). Women have access to specialised care for more complex needs and a dedicated area for those who want non-pharmacological methods for pain relief, water birth, freedom to adopt any position during labour and delivery, one-to-one midwifery care and privacy. Nagela describes 'a warm and welcoming environment' that contrasts with the normalised obstetric violence in other Brazilian hospitals.

Services, campaigners, feminists and policymakers need to address the individual in front of them. Feminists looking at birth must ensure their focus is on the individual, looking outwards at how, when the voice of that individual isn't heard, our broader rights are threatened at the most fundamental level.

Pregnancy as a crime

US resident Bei Bei Shuai was eight months pregnant when she discovered that her boyfriend was already married and abandoning her that day to rejoin his 'real' family in China. Devastated, she decided to end her life. Emergency hospital treatment saved her but Shuai's baby sadly died in her arms after only four days of life. It took only 30 minutes for the homicide branch to send a detective to the hospital to question staff. Two and a half months later, Shuai was charged with murder and 'feticide' under Indiana state law. She served more than a year in a high-security prison without bail and, once bailed, the state surveyed her movements via an electronic tag. She eventually pleaded guilty to a lesser charge of criminal recklessness after flaws in the prosecution's evidence were exposed and the original charges were dropped.

Cases of women being criminalised because they are pregnant are easy to dismiss as aberrations but, en masse, they are harder to ignore. In 2013, the National Advocates for Pregnant Women (NAPW) published a study identifying 413 arrests and forced interventions on pregnant women between 1973 and 2005.[80] Since 2005 they have identified a further 380, with more arrests each week. Cases include women being arrested and charged with murder or feticide after miscarriages and stillbirths, court-ordered imprisonment in hospital following premature labour, and arrests for drinking alcohol in pregnancy. In one case, a woman who moved states while pregnant was accused of 'appropriating the child whilst in utero' by the custodial court and told to return to the state the child's father resided in. Lynn Paltrow of NAPW points to a direct link between this massive upswing in punitive measures for pregnant women and what the Guttmacher Institute describes as a 'seismic shift' in the number of US states using legal measures to restrict or remove the right to abortion.[81]

Every major health organisation in America opposes criminalising women for the outcome of their pregnancies. Yet on 3 February 2015 the latest victim of politically motivated prosecutions stood in front of a jury in an Indiana court room. They took just six hours to convict 33-year-old Purvi Patel of 'feticide' and child neglect. Astonishingly, although the charges were entirely contradictory (the first conviction rested on proving the foetus was born dead, and the second that it was born living) she was convicted of both. Patel maintains she suffered a stillbirth and in panic and shock left her dead baby behind a dumpster, presenting later at the emergency room with pain and bleeding. Yet, despite no evidence of drugs in her system, state prosecutors maintained she had used illegal abortion medication to induce labour deliberately. There has been widespread condemnation of the case from medical experts, human rights activists and women's rights groups, but Patel has now been sentenced to 20 years in prison. This in a state that makes free, safe abortion as difficult and as emotionally painful as possible.

In November 2014 voters in Colorado were asked to consider 'amendment 67' on a state-wide ballot. It was the third time a 'personhood' amendment had come before them and once again it was defeated, with 34 per cent of voters in support. However, many of us believe it is only a matter of time before a similar amendment is passed somewhere in the US. Until then, at least 38 other US states[82] now have 'feticide' laws that, like the defeated Colorado amendment, have been introduced in the wake of violence against pregnant women and are dressed up as ways to protect them and their unborn children.

Heather Surovik was eight months pregnant in July 2012 when a drunk driver crashed into her car, injuring her and killing her unborn son, Brady. Since his tragic death she has campaigned for a change to the Colorado state law to enable future drivers to be criminally prosecuted for death of the unborn. Her motivation is understandable. The amendment was a deceptively simple one, asking that the words 'person' and 'child' in both Colorado's Criminal Code and its Wrongful Death Act should now include unborn human beings; fertilised eggs, embryos and foetuses that a woman carries within her body.

Significantly heavier penalties for those who perpetrate violence against pregnant women, as enacted around the world, are the appropriate way to acknowledge these horrific tragedies and the harm they can cause. However, foetal personhood and 'feticide' laws are far more ambitious than that. In Colorado, by altering the definition of the words 'person' and 'child', abortion would be made first-degree murder. It could lead to the widespread imprisonment of women experiencing stillbirths and miscarriages, and more women having court-ordered interventions like caesarean sections against their will. Women who drink or smoke or otherwise fall foul of arbitrary guidelines could be prosecuted for their actions, whether or not they can be shown to have caused direct harm to the child.

Slippery slope arguments are unpopular, but here the incursions into women's freedoms are not theoretical. The 380 cases NAPW has documented since 2005 are testament to that and include examples of all of the above. Worryingly, none of the 38 states that have passed 'feticide' laws have done any research to determine whether they have reduced violence against pregnant women or protected them in any way. Research has demonstrated, however, that these laws have been used repeatedly to arrest pregnant women. Individual campaigners may be misguidedly seeking to protect women via these laws, but those who write them and fund the campaigns do not have women's best interests at heart. Instead, they seize on individual tragedy, using its emotive power to undermine the rights women have fought hard to achieve.

Are we next? UK criminalisation

As I've shown above, the highest UK courts have defended women's rights to autonomy when challenged, but 2014 saw a frightening legal attack on women's reproductive rights in the UK.

In September 2014 Birthrights and the British Pregnancy Advisory Service made a written intervention[83] in the English Court of Appeal hearing of CP v Criminal Injuries Compensation Authority. This case sought compensation for a child born with foetal alcohol spectrum disorder (FASD), which stemmed from her alcoholic mother's drinking during pregnancy. While both charities felt that the child should be afforded the specialised state help with education that the compensation sought to cover, we felt this wasn't the way to guarantee it. Moreover, we were concerned that this test case would set a legal precedent that could compromise the freedom of pregnant women's rights more broadly.

Media and public interest in the case was intense. Criticisms of the proposal were heavily focused on the counterproductive nature of criminal penalties and the risk of driving vulnerable women away from help, alongside the disproportionate penalisation of vulnerable groups, such as women with mental health problems, victims of domestic abuse and those at the lowest end of the socioeconomic scale.

Yet some commentators' arguments were worryingly similar to those of the 'vote yes' to the Colorado amendment 67 campaign. They focused on getting 'justice' for the individual struck by tragedy or injury and insisted there would be no wider implications. What was not written about was the interest of the anti-abortion movement in the case.

The Pro-Life Research Unit (PRU), funded by the Right to Life Charitable Trust, CARE and LIFE, also intervened. In their intervention, they are keen to dismiss the possibilities of a precedent set in the CP case leading to future prosecutions of pregnant women. However, the US example demonstrates how swiftly any chink in the legal armour around women's rights to make decisions about their bodies during pregnancy is accessed by the anti-abortion movement.

The PRU's intervention makes assertions that disprove their claim that this case is about individual compensation. Stating in it that 'it seems uncontroversial that the foetus is human, possesses at least some of the attributes of personhood and is entitled to protection in the name of human dignity', the PRU also makes contentions which they acknowledge are beyond the scope of this case. They ask that domestic courts determine issues of foetal personhood and whether a foetus has Article 2 or Article 8 rights under the 1998 Human Rights Act. It reads strategically as a first step to challenging abortion in the UK.

I believe the PRU's intervention is an almost inevitable attempt by the anti-abortion lobby to replicate their US colleagues' strategic claiming of pregnancy. Lynn Paltrow describes the well-funded expert operation in the US, where those drafting 'feticide' and foetal personhood laws have a 'long-term, deliberate strategy that's absolutely traceable'. Judges like Alabama Supreme Court Justice Tom Parker,[84] who has spoken very publicly about his anti-abortion stance, has a history of using legal cases to further the anti-abortion movement. Tragic stories, such as the prosecution of Hope Ankrom after her newborn son tested positive for cocaine and marijuana, have legally undermined a woman's capacity to control what happens to her body when she becomes pregnant, with no demonstrable benefit to future children born to drug-addicted mothers. The strategy is to repeatedly confer more weight on the rights of the foetus in cases connected with pregnancy and birth, rather than focus on abortion itself. This sustained campaign, Paltrow states, seeks to 'pass as many laws as possible to give the foetus rights as a basis for overturning Roe'. The Roe v Wade case, which precipitated legal abortion in America, is, Paltrow believes, vulnerable at the moment, and exploitation of weak links in pregnancy and birth-related rights have played a vital part in making it so.

When asked about the PRU's intervention in the CP case in England, Paltrow is emphatic in her agreement with my belief that this marks a major initial step in a broader strategic campaign to undermine women's essential human dignity and limit their access to abortion. 'The US is always exporting its worst policies,' she asserts, 'and you can feel very confident that this is part of a bigger strategy. It is very obvious. There's no doubt.'

The impact of this broader strategy and the pervasiveness of a mother vs foetus view is far-reaching. In November 2015 Essex woman Lauren Bull awoke to discover a pool of blood in her bed after suffering stomach cramps for the past two days. Unaware she was pregnant, Lauren went on to miscarry a 18–22 week foetus in the family bathroom. Worried about frightening their two children, Lauren and partner Jack Walker cleaned the bathroom and then went to hospital. It is unclear exactly why the police were called or who called them, but a forensic team were sent to the house and staggeringly the couple were charged with murder the following day.

Despite the trauma of her miscarriage, Lauren and her partner were forced to spend the night in police custody before the charge was downgraded to 'concealing the birth of a child' and the couple were released. The current status of their potential prosecution is unknown. Though the circumstances in Lauren's case are highly unusual, it illustrates the vulnerability of pregnant women even in England, where the legal position should prevent miscarriage leading to a murder charge.

A few hundred miles away in Ireland the picture for women is very different. The 1983 eighth amendment to the Irish constitution added Article 40.3.3, which reads:

> The State acknowledges the right to life of the unborn and, with due regard to the equal right to life of the mother, guarantees in its laws to respect, and, as far as practicable, by its laws to defend and vindicate that right.

Introduced to ensure Ireland did not follow the lead of America and England and legalise abortion in any circumstance, the amendment stands to this day despite vigorous campaigning.

In January 2016 a new pro-choice group launched, explicitly making the link between the need to repeal the eighth amendment to give Irish women the right to abortion and also to ensure autonomy in childbirth. Speaking as Midwives for Choice (MfC) launched, midwife and MfC activist Philomena Canning explained the link:

> ...the eighth amendment has failed in its objective of fetal protection from abortion. While undermining the human rights of women by denying access to safe, free and legal abortion in Ireland, the eighth amendment also has damning implications for choice across the spectrum of pregnancy and childbirth, evidenced by its exclusion of all pregnant women from the National Consent Policy.

The National Consent Policy was adopted across Ireland in 2014 with the explicit purpose of providing a single, unified policy outlining consent in Irish law and how it should be interpreted in healthcare. The introduction explains that the 'ethical rationale behind the importance of consent is the need to respect the service user's right to self-determination (or autonomy) – their right to control their own life and to decide what happens to their own body.'[85]

A short paragraph on consent in pregnancy makes it clear how the eighth amendment has removed women's right to autonomy:

> ...because of the constitutional provisions on the right to life of the 'unborn', there is significant legal uncertainty regarding the extent of a pregnant woman's right to refuse treatment in circumstances in which the refusal would put the life of a viable foetus at serious risk. In such circumstances, legal advice should be sought as to whether an application to the High Court is necessary.

The death of Savita Halappanavar in Galway in 2012 following a miscarriage serves as a reminder of how brutally clinicians and courts have interpreted the legal position. They chose to privilege the rights of an unviable foetus above the bodily autonomy of the woman carrying it, despite her repeated requests for a termination. The inquest into her death returned a verdict of 'medical misadventure', recommending that the Irish Medical Council lay out new guidelines on when doctors can intervene to save the life of a mother.

Philomena Canning believes that denying women a role in decision-making about their care in pregnancy and childbirth undermines the safety and welfare of mothers and babies. She notes the link between an anti-abortion rhetoric and the safety of birthing women too:

> *...in the name of fetal protectionism, the eighth amendment provides for the enforced compliance of healthy women in childbirth with routine intervention – without medical necessity and contrary to best practice.*

We mustn't be complacent about our reproductive rights, even in England where it can at first appear that we have little to worry about. As the ongoing 'We Trust Women' campaign reminds us, abortion has still not been decriminalised even in a country that is overwhelming pro-choice. As women in Ireland and the US have experienced, it is all too easy to use the law punitively and restrictively against women's freedoms. It is essential that we continue to expose anti-women agendas in the courtroom and political arena and campaign for them to be reversed. We must also robustly defend and promote women's rights in childbirth to ensure they are not a weak point in our reproductive armour.

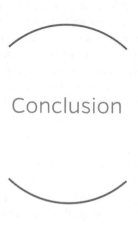

Conclusion

I could write you a book about my first birth but this one was just so simple. I could not believe the difference from last time. I actually felt happy to be holding my baby – an experience utterly denied me with my first child. More than this, experiencing the second birth on my terms has made me happier and a more confident mother to my son, too. If I had to describe this birth in one word (even though everyone says childbirth is magic, a miracle) the word for this would be: straightforward. Blessedly, wonderfully so.

I was there when Anne gave birth on her own terms. She smiled and held her daughter, looking shocked and relieved. It doesn't make for an exciting story, but after the traumatic forceps birth that left her physically and emotionally damaged for at least a year, this time she needed a different kind of care in a different kind of system. She was able to access case-loading midwifery via her local NHS trust. An out-of-hospital birth matched her needs and with it came an awareness of her right to ask questions, make decisions and be treated as an individual.

A good birth is not rocket science and birth can be positive even if it doesn't go to plan. For many women, though, it slips through their fingers due to a basic lack of maternity services or the industrialised, technocratic systems that contain them. Attitudes to women in general, and mothering and birth specifically, and the often shaky understanding or flagrant abuse of human rights, also stand between them and the simple pursuit of straightforward childbirth. One that reflects their humanity, is as safe as possible for them and their babies, and leaves them feeling as emotionally robust as they did before.

For this to happen, a fundamental change in the dichotomised presentation of birth and mothering is required. We need to reframe it as something that happens to individual women rather than a political or moral act. The 'women's business' of Indigenous Australian culture is perhaps a very apt term. Rather than a rhetorical mismatch between ideas of 'woman-centred' care and the reality of a system toxic to the women at its centre, policymakers, commissioners and those training healthcare providers must also make a dignified, respectful and compassionate approach to maternity care a reality.

As I look around the landscape of birth today, I can see that grassroots and top-down action over the past two years in human rights and childbirth is beginning to make progress towards these goals. There's a palpable energy around applying these tools to birth. The White Ribbon Alliance's charter of rights (which sets out seven rights every woman should expect to be upheld in the maternity system)[86] is being implemented across the world from Nepal to Barking. At the same time, organisations like Human Rights in Childbirth and Birthrights are driving forward initiatives like the publication of a free human rights guide for midwives, funded by the UK's

Equality and Human Rights Commission. Birthrights will be providing free and paid-for-training on respectful care to midwives and doctors around the UK on a bigger scale, while Human Rights in Childbirth is reaching out globally with summits in India, America, Eastern Europe and Africa.

Although on the surface it hardly seems like the stuff of revolution, in late 2014 the National Institute for Health and Care Excellence (NICE) published updated guidelines[87] on caring for women in labour, which could fan these sparks of change. These guidelines should, in theory, inform the practice of all those caring for labouring women in the UK. The new version makes some radical departures from the past. Most widely reported was the insistence that all women should be presented with quality evidence about where to give birth, directing healthcare professionals to put their personal feelings on the matter aside. For low-risk women, evidence showed that out-of-hospital, midwife-led care was most appropriate, though NICE urged that all options should be available to women. Less reported, but more interesting to me, was the focus throughout on dignity. My favourite line urges commissioners and staff to

...ensure that there is a culture of respect for each woman as an individual undergoing a significant and emotionally intense life experience, so that the woman is in control, is listened to and is cared for with compassion, and that appropriate informed consent is sought.

Looking ahead, if these guidelines become more than words on paper, they could usher in a positive new era of maternity care in the UK. The challenge, of course, will be to ensure they are not simply more rhetoric that contributes to women feeling guilty and confused about the real experience they have within an unfriendly system.

A day after the NICE guidelines were published, on 4 December 2014, Court of Appeal judges ruled on the CP v Criminal Injuries Compensation Authority case, dismissing the appeal and affirming that the state should fund appropriate specialist care for children affected by foetal alcohol spectrum disorders (FASD) without criminalising their mothers. If the US example is anything to go by, we can expect more challenges of this nature, but matching the tangible opportunity this presents to the anti-abortion movement is an important chance for us to resist the tide of censure that is engulfing pregnant women. We can be encouraged that this case demonstrates that UK courts and public opinion support the idea that women must remain at the helm of their reproductive futures. That neither they nor their future children are well served by making them criminals.

It's also an opportunity to insist on support services for vulnerable women so that they are able to control substance abuse problems during pregnancy and less likely to end up in the complex and often horrific circumstances that make them unable to discharge their responsibilities as pregnant women. This is emphatically not, as some critics like anti-abortion peer Lord Deben have suggested, about throwing unborn children 'on the scrapheap'. Turning this argument into a battle between woman and foetus just isn't a realistic interpretation of the realities of pregnancy. Children with additional needs require specialist care. It is ridiculous to suggest that a criminal compensation scheme, also funded by a public pot, is the only way to provide them with this.

Legal structures, challenges and policies across the world are recognising women's rights in birth. In 2013, thanks to the work of the White Ribbon Alliance, the Nepalese government promised to include women's right to respectful maternity care in law. The Brazilian government has invested over 4 million dollars in the 'Stork Network' – part of the National Public Health System. This network of care stems from the grassroots 'humanising birth movement' that reaches across South America. The movement has been successful in garnering national governmental support in addition to World Health Organization assistance. The Stork Network aims to ensure women's rights to reproductive planning and humanised care during pregnancy, childbirth and the postpartum period are met. Importantly, the network places emphasis on accessibility of abortion and looks at children and babies' rights as interdependent with those of their mothers.[88]

Here in England the National Maternity Review published in 2016 made rights-respecting care a key part of its vision. The team tried to end the safety v choice debate, stating that 'safe maternity care is personalised care', and insisting that genuine choice and unbiased information should be supported by healthcare professionals and service infrastructure. Seven pilot areas have been chosen to offer personalised maternity budgets. Though the details of the scheme are still being worked out, pregnant people in these regions will be able to choose who provides their antenatal, birth and postnatal care, at least theoretically ensuring that choice of place of birth is a reality for all. In this and a number of other significant ways, the review provides yet another tool in advancing the respectful care agenda in the UK.

For me, one of the most significant opportunities that is suddenly at our disposal (in addition to systemic and cultural changes) is the growing realisation that a women's rights agenda has to be fought collectively. Clare Murphy of bpas describes an increasing awareness that the rights of all women are best served by looking at health and reproductive rights as interdependent. She explains that 'they need to rest on the principle that women are the ones best placed to make decisions about their bodies and their births', adding that 'we will really be on to something if we join forces and start to look at these issues together'.

Murphy and I believe that we are talking about the same women, and that the woman who has an abortion or miscarriage is the very same one who births a baby and feeds him. Undermining one aspect of her reproductive freedom, whether it is where or how she gives birth or if she can safely have an abortion, inevitably has knock-on consequences for the others. Across the board there's a need to give women the evidence and trust them to make their own choices. With those choices comes great responsibility, and we must do all that we can to ensure that women are in circumstances that allow them to exercise that responsibility appropriately. For the very rare few who can't or won't, the uncomfortable and sometimes tragic reality is that there may be consequences for her and her baby. This is hard to accept and we must do all we can to avoid it, offering state support when it does happen, without throwing aside the broader rights of women in pursuit of an impossible goal.

Lynn Paltrow, speaking from the US where women are increasingly unable to exercise their basic reproductive freedoms, agrees. Despite the hostile climate towards women, she feels that suddenly 'people are listening in a way they haven't before', but that if reverse progress continues unchecked, abortion could all too soon become illegal throughout the country. Yet, as more incursions into women's reproductive rights are made, they become harder for us to ignore. Rather than being the end of the road, Paltrow feels that if Roe v Wade is overturned it will be the beginning. She sounds tired, frightened, yet full of hope when she affirms that a removal of legal abortion in the US 'will ignite a political movement by women the likes of which has never been seen'.

When I look at my six-year-old daughter I wonder what the world will look like when she comes to make these choices about her health and body. Will her reproductive rights be more or less protected than mine? Will the myth of 'a healthy baby is all that matters' have been unpicked? Will it all matter and will human rights have helped to get us there? I hope so. By then I hope this book will be a dusty anachronism, but I know that if not, she and her contemporaries will continue to fight for it.

Women are powerful. If childbirth (in its many forms) teaches us one thing, it is that.

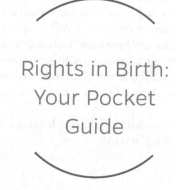

Rights in Birth: Your Pocket Guide

The information in this guide is taken from the Birthrights factsheets on human rights in childbirth available at birthrights.org.uk. The guidance applies to women in England, Scotland and Wales, but should not be used in place of legal or medical advice.

If you are outside these countries please see the Resources and Further Reading section for details of how to find support and information in your area.

Rights in brief

- Every woman has a right to receive safe and appropriate maternity care.
- Every woman has a right to maternity care that respects her fundamental human dignity.
- Every woman has a right to privacy and confidentiality.
- Every woman is free to make choices about her own pregnancy and childbirth, even if her caregivers do not agree with her.

- Every woman has a right to equality and freedom from discrimination.

Human rights and maternity care: an overview

Human rights law gives pregnant women the right to receive maternity care; to make their own choices about their care; and to be given standards of care that respect their dignity as human beings.

What are human rights?

Every human being has human rights. Human rights protect your dignity, your privacy, your equality and your autonomy (your control over your own life). Human rights require public bodies to treat you with dignity, consult you about certain decisions and respect your choices.

Where do human rights come from?

Human rights in Europe are protected by the European Convention on Human Rights. The Convention sets out the minimum rights that all European countries have to respect. In the UK, the European Convention rights have been incorporated into law by the Human Rights Act 1998. This means that if a person thinks they have been denied their rights under theg Convention, they can bring a legal claim in the UK courts. The UK has also ratified the Convention on the Elimination of Discrimination Against Women, which prohibits pregnancy-related discrimination and requires the provision of healthcare for pregnant and lactating women. The Convention influences the UK courts' interpretation of the law, but it is not possible to bring a legal claim under the Convention.

Why are human rights relevant to maternity care?

The fundamental human rights values of dignity, privacy, equality and autonomy are often relevant to the way a woman is treated during pregnancy and childbirth. Failure to provide adequate maternity care, lack of respect for women's dignity, invasions of privacy, procedures carried out without consent, failure to provide adequate pain relief without medical contraindication, giving pain relief where it is not requested, unnecessary or unexplained medical interventions, and lack of respect for women's choices about where and how a birth takes place, may all violate human rights and can lead to women feeling degraded and dehumanised.

How do human rights apply to maternity care?

Under the Human Rights Act, all UK public bodies must respect the rights set out in the European Convention. Public bodies include all NHS institutions, such as hospitals, Primary Care Trusts, NHS Trusts and Clinical Commissioning Groups. This means that public bodies must respect human rights when making decisions. It also means that caregivers working in public bodies must respect human rights as they go about their work.

Do I have a right to receive maternity care?

Yes. All pregnant women in the UK have a right to receive maternity care. Although the European Convention does not explicitly guarantee a right to healthcare, Article 2 protects the right to life and requires the state to provide access to basic life-saving health services, including maternity care. Overseas citizens may be charged for maternity care in some circumstances, but care must be provided regardless of whether the patient can pay the charge. See pages 152-155 for more information.

Do I have a right to make choices about my care?

Yes. Women have the right to make their own choices about how they manage their pregnancy and birth. Article 8 of the European Convention guarantees the right to private life, which the courts have interpreted to include the right to physical autonomy and integrity.

The right to autonomy means that a woman's consent must always be sought before performing any medical procedure on her. Failure to obtain consent violates Article 8, and may also violate the prohibition on inhuman and degrading treatment under Article 3. Failure to provide sufficient, objective and unbiased information for a woman to make an informed choice will also violate Article 8. See pages 136-144 for more information on consenting to treatment. The European Court of Human Rights has held that the right to private life includes a right for women to make choices about the circumstances in which they give birth, including whether to give birth at home (Ternovszky v Hungary, 2011). See pages 45 for more information. The right to make choices about childbirth includes the right to refuse any medical care at all. See pages 155 for more information on unassisted birth.

Do human rights guarantee standards of care?

Yes. All women are entitled to care that respects their basic dignity, privacy and autonomy. Article 3 of the European Convention prohibits inhuman and degrading treatment. If caregivers fail to provide care that is needed to avoid preventable suffering – such as pain relief – then this can amount to inhuman or degrading treatment. Article 8 of the European Convention, as interpreted by the courts, requires public bodies to respect dignity and autonomy.

Article 14 of the European Convention prohibits discrimination and entitles women to equal treatment in their maternity care. This makes it unlawful for NHS organisations or individual caregivers to discriminate against pregnant women on irrelevant grounds such as disability, race, religion, immigration status and national origin.

Do human rights protect an unborn child?

No. Unborn children do not have separate legal recognition under the European Convention or in the common law of England and Wales. Women are free to make choices against medical advice and cannot be forced to accept treatment which is said to be in the unborn child's interest. See pages 136-144 for more information on consenting to treatment.

If healthcare providers believe that a woman is putting her baby at risk they may make a referral to social services, which have the power to make a child protection plan for an unborn child. However, the threat of referral to social services should never be used to intimidate, bully or coerce a woman into accepting a particular medical intervention for her or her child. Consent that is given on the basis of such a threat is not given freely, and the health professional may be legally liable for battery and violation of Article 8 of the European Convention if they perform the intervention and they know, or should know, that consent has not been freely given.

Consenting to treatment

Pregnant women – like everyone else – have the right to make their own decisions about their bodies. It is against the law to give medical treatment to a pregnant woman unless she agrees to it. This is known legally as giving her consent.

Basic principles

Every person has the right to make decisions about their body for themselves. This is known as the principle of autonomy. It is protected under the common law of England and Wales and Article 8 of the European Convention on Human Rights. Pregnant women are entitled to make autonomous decisions in the same way as any other person, and their decisions must be respected, regardless of whether health professionals agree with them. The principle of autonomy creates a legal requirement to obtain a person's consent whenever they are given any medical treatment. The only exceptions to this are in rare cases: either when a person does not have the capacity to make their own decisions; or in an emergency when a person cannot consent because of their physical condition.

If a person's consent is not obtained, the medical treatment will be against the law on several counts. It will constitute the crime of battery, and a civil wrong of trespass to the person and/or negligence, and it will violate Article 8 of the European Convention. If the harm that occurs as a result is serious, it will also breach Article 3 of the European Convention prohibiting inhuman and degrading treatment.

When is consent required?

Consent is required for every medical procedure. Consent must be obtained before any examination or investigation is carried out, or any care or treatment is provided. The fact that a woman has consented to a particular procedure in the past does not mean that she consents automatically to the same procedure again. Consent must be sought each time a procedure is performed. If circumstances change or new information becomes available, and the benefits or risks of the treatment change as a result, then fresh consent should be sought. Sometimes, a healthcare professional may ask for advance consent to treat problems that could arise while the woman is unable to give further consent. For this reason, consent forms for caesarean section will often list other procedures which the woman is asked to 'pre-authorise', in case they should become necessary during the operation and the woman is unable to give her consent because she is under general anaesthetic or lacks capacity. Any procedure not mentioned on the form may only be carried out if it will prevent death or serious harm.

What counts as consent?

For consent to 'count' in the law, a person must genuinely agree to receive treatment. This means that the woman must be well-enough informed about the treatment, and cannot have been put under undue pressure or bullied into receiving the treatment by healthcare professionals or family members. These requirements are explained in detail below.

What information should I be given?

You must be given information about any proposed procedure in advance. The information should cover any significant risks, any alternative treatments which are available, and the risks of doing nothing. However, the law does not require that doctors and midwives give women all the information within their knowledge. They must provide enough information so that the general nature and purpose of the treatment is properly understood.

Giving misleading information about your medical condition or the proposed treatment, or not giving you relevant information, may mean that consent was not valid. The failure to provide appropriate information may also leave the healthcare professional open to a successful claim of negligence where the woman suffers harm as a result of the treatment.

If a woman asks specific questions, it is good practice for a healthcare professional to give full, honest and objective answers. The GMC guidance advises doctors to encourage their patients to ask questions. The healthcare professional regulators, the General Medical Council (GMC) and the Nursing and Midwifery Council (NMC), produce guidance on consent, explaining in detail what information doctors and midwives are expected to provide, as well as how consent should be recorded. The Royal College of Obstetricians and Gynaecologists also provides advice on consent, and on specific procedures and the risks associated with those procedures, including caesarean section, operative vaginal delivery, and participating in research while in labour.

What is undue pressure?

A healthcare professional must explain the risks of a procedure to a woman, including risks to her unborn child, and may recommend a particular clinical option. However, they must not put 'undue pressure' on the woman to accept their advice. 'Undue pressure' could include physical restraint, threats to withdraw care, repetitive and unwanted discussion of risks, imposing an arbitrary time limit for a decision, and putting pressure on other family members.

A threat to refer a woman to social services would constitute undue pressure. Such a threat should never be used to intimidate, bully or coerce a woman into accepting a particular medical procedure for her or her unborn child. Consent that is given on this basis may not constitute valid consent, and the healthcare professional may be legally liable if they performed the medical intervention.

Should consent be recorded in writing?

Consent does not need to be recorded in writing. Consent

may be given verbally or even with a gesture, for example by holding out your arm for blood pressure to be checked. It is usual practice to sign a consent form for surgical procedures.

Where there has been a discussion about a procedure, the medical records should include details of the discussion, including information given and any questions asked by the patient. A signed consent form and/or medical notes are evidence of consent but not proof: they may be contradicted by other evidence that consent was not well-enough informed or freely given. The GMC's guidance and Department of Health's reference guide contain further information on the form consent should take.

What happens in an emergency?

In an emergency, the general principle is that if a patient is unable to make their wishes known, treatment can be given without their consent in order to save their life or prevent serious deterioration in their condition. If there is time, the patient's next-of-kin should be involved in decisions about their care.

Can I refuse treatment?

Yes. The English courts have upheld the rights of patients 'to make important medical decisions affecting their lives for themselves: they have the right to make decisions which doctors regard as ill advised' (Re MB (Adult, medical treatment), 1997). A mentally competent patient has an absolute right to refuse medical treatment for any reason, rational or irrational, or for no reason at all, even where that decision may lead to his or her own death. A mentally competent woman may refuse treatment even where that might lead to death or serious harm to her or her baby (St George's Healthcare NHS Trust v S, 1997).

The Royal College of Obstetricians and Gynaecologists' ethics committee guideline on court-authorised caesarean section provides further details on the very limited circumstances in which the court can authorise caesarean sections.

Can I withdraw consent?

Yes. Once given, consent remains valid for the relevant procedure unless it is withdrawn. Consent can be withdrawn at any time. It may not always be possible to stop a procedure immediately, but if the healthcare professional has any doubts about whether a woman has withdrawn her consent, they should stop as soon as possible and check whether or not she still consents.

What is mental capacity?

It is always assumed that a woman has the mental capacity to consent to treatment (or to refuse it) unless it can be shown otherwise. This principle is enshrined in the Mental Capacity Act 2005, which governs decisions about whether a person lacks capacity and how they can be treated if they do.

In order to lack capacity under the law, a woman must be unable to make a decision for herself because of a problem in the functioning of her mind. She might lack capacity in relation to some decisions and not others. The fact that a woman may have made a seemingly irrational decision that clinicians believe is not in her best interests is not a reason by itself to decide that she lacks capacity. If a woman is deemed to lack capacity, decisions about her treatment must be made in her best interests. The Mental Capacity Act sets out the factors that should be taken into account in deciding someone's best interests. This includes taking account of any written statement of preferences or wishes, which could include a birth plan.

Where there is serious doubt or dispute about a person's capacity or best interests, the Court of Protection can be asked to make a ruling. It may make a binding decision regarding treatment or may appoint a deputy to make decisions on behalf of the patient.

The Mental Capacity Act 2005 Code of Practice gives further detail on how the Mental Capacity Act should be applied. If a woman is being treated for a mental disorder under the Mental Health Act 1983, that does not necessarily mean that she lacks capacity in relation to decisions about her maternity care. She should be treated in the same way as any other woman unless she has been assessed to lack capacity.

Will giving birth affect my capacity to consent?

Extremely rarely. The experience of giving birth will not affect whether you have capacity to consent to treatment, except in very exceptional circumstances where capacity is completely destroyed by drugs, fatigue, pain or anxiety. Royal College of Obstetricians and Gynaecologists' guidance and guidance on consent from the Association of Anaesthetists of Great Britain and Northern Ireland state that special care must be taken when obtaining consent from women who are in labour, particularly if they are under the influence of narcotic analgesics (opiate-derived painkilling drugs).

What happens if I lose capacity?

If you suffer from a condition that may cause you to lose capacity during your pregnancy or labour, you could make an 'advance decision' about your maternity treatment under the Mental Capacity Act 2005. An advance decision will have the same effect as a decision made in labour and must be followed by healthcare professionals. This advance decision can be withdrawn at any time.

An advance decision must meet certain criteria set out in the Mental Capacity Act 2005. It must, for example, make it clear which treatments the person is refusing and it must be signed and witnessed. If an advance decision refuses life-sustaining treatment when life is at risk, it must clearly state this.

An advance decision cannot request specific medical treatment, it can only refuse treatments. A written statement of wishes or preferences, such as a birth plan, which does not qualify as an advance decision under the act, does not legally bind a healthcare professional like an advance decision would. However, it should be used to guide any decisions if a woman loses capacity.

What is the legal status of a birth plan?

A birth plan is a statement of a woman's preferred plan of care during labour and postnatally. It does not have any formal legal status, but it ought to be respected by healthcare professionals unless the woman gives her consent to a different plan of care. A birth plan may be used as evidence of consent or lack of consent if a woman later challenges the treatment that she has received. If treatment that a woman has requested in her birth plan is clinically contraindicated (i.e. there are medical reasons for not providing the treatment), she should be told the reasons for refusing to provide the treatment.

Healthcare providers have a duty to prevent avoidable suffering, so refusal of pain relief, access to a birth pool or other forms of support during labour should be considered with reference to each woman's individual circumstances and not solely on the basis of a guideline or policy.

Can I decide what treatment my baby receives?

Yes. Consent for any medical treatment or procedure, including the administration of a drug, must be sought from a person with 'parental responsibility' for the baby. This always includes the baby's mother, although the baby's father has parental responsibility only if certain criteria are met. You can find a summary of parental responsibility on the NHS Choices website. If parents refuse treatment for their child, healthcare professionals should respect their decision. In some circumstances, including if parents disagree about treatment, healthcare professionals may approach the High Court for an order declaring that treatment is in a child's best interests and should be carried out.

Choice of place of birth

Can I choose where to give birth?

Yes. The law protects your right to decide where you give birth. The legal principle of consent means that you cannot be compelled to give birth in any particular location or medical setting against your will, so long as you have mental capacity to make your own decisions.

Do I have a right to choose hospital care?

Yes. All women in the UK are entitled to maternity care in hospital. In some circumstances, women who are not resident in the UK will be charged for their care, but it cannot be withheld from them if they cannot pay. See p.152 for information on foreign nationals and maternity care.

Do I have a right to out-of-hospital services?

All NHS Trusts are expected by the Department of Health to make out-of-hospital services available to women in their area. According to Department of Health guidance issued to the NHS, women's choice of place of birth, whether in hospital, in a birth centre or at home, should be a 'national choice guarantee'.

However, there remains regional variation in the out-of-hospital services available to women. Article 8 of the European

Convention on Human Rights protects every person's right to respect for their autonomous choice about their private life. In Ternovszky v Hungary, 2010, the European Court found that this includes women's right to decide the circumstances, and location, in which they give birth. Article 8 is a qualified right. Respect for private life and autonomous choices can be limited only if there are genuinely legitimate reasons for doing so and these are proportionate. But the public body refusing to respect a person's choice would have to prove the reasons for limiting choice, and show that these were proportionate. If an NHS Trust refuses to provide a home birth service, this may breach your Article 8 rights unless it can give good reasons for its decision, which must be backed up by evidence.

If you have been told by your midwife or other healthcare professionals during your pregnancy that you can give birth at home or in a birth centre, you may have a 'legitimate expectation' of giving birth there. This is simply a legal way of saying that you should get what you have been promised. It is only lawful to refuse to honour a legitimate expectation if there are proportionate reasons for doing so.

If staffing shortages are given as a reason for refusing your choice of place of birth, a hospital may be expected to have contingency plans in place (such as hiring independent midwives) to ensure that there are enough staff to provide the services it has promised.

If an NHS Trust does not offer birth centre facilities, you ought to be able to access a birth centre in a neighbouring area. You can ask your GP for a referral at any point in your pregnancy.

Are midwives obliged to attend home births?

Midwives are under a professional obligation to respect a woman's decision to give birth outside hospital and attend a woman at home if requested, regardless of whether they agree with a woman's choice. The Nursing and Midwifery Council has issued guidance which states:

- Midwives have a 'duty of care' to attend women at home.
- Any midwife who withdraws care from a woman will be held professionally accountable for their decision. This means the midwife could face disciplinary sanctions by the Nursing and Midwifery Council for failing to attend a home birth.
- Local Supervising Authority midwifery officers, supervisors of midwives and midwifery managers have a professional duty to support midwives to provide home births. If a healthcare professional has breached their duty of care, they can be referred to their regulatory body.

Can I still give birth at home if I am 'high-risk'?

You are responsible for making your decisions about where you give birth. Your decision cannot lawfully be overridden by anyone else, unless you lack mental capacity to make decisions about your healthcare.

If you are advised against giving birth at home, you cannot be compelled to attend hospital. Your midwife and hospital consultant, if you have one, should work with you to put in place a care plan that makes it possible for you to exercise your choice to give birth at home. The midwife may also involve her supervisor of midwives in planning your care. Healthcare professionals must present information about birth choices in an unbiased and objective way.

If a woman has made a decision in response to coercion or threats, including the threat of involvement of social services, she may not have given her consent to treatment, and the healthcare professional may be legally liable for failing to obtain consent.

Your right to medical assistance

Am I entitled to receive obstetric care?

As a result of the serious and occasionally life-threatening health complications that can occur in pregnancy and childbirth, all women are entitled to access to medical attention from an obstetrician and/or gynaecologist.

Article 2 of the European Convention on Human Rights protects the right to life and requires the state to provide access to basic life-saving health services, which include maternity care in hospital. If you have a complication in your pregnancy, or you have a reason for concern about your pregnancy or birth, you should be given the opportunity to consult an obstetrician.

Do I have a right to pain relief?

You have a right to make informed choices about the circumstances in which you give birth for yourself. If you have requested pain relief, it should be provided unless there are good reasons for refusing to provide it, such as a clinical contraindication (i.e. a medical reason for not providing the treatment).

Article 3 of the European Convention prohibits inhuman and degrading treatment. If caregivers fail to provide care which is needed to avoid preventable suffering – such as pain relief in a clinically appropriate form – then this could amount to inhuman or degrading treatment in some circumstances, such as undergoing procedures without appropriate anaesthetic.

Caesarean sections

What if there's a clinical need for a caesarean section?

If there is a clinical need to perform a c-section, it must be made available in an appropriate time scale. Failure to perform a c-section could constitute medical negligence. Where there is a threat to the life of mother or child, hospitals and individual clinicians are obliged to take steps to save life under Article 2 of the European Convention on Human Rights, enacted in UK law by the Human Rights Act 1998.

Maternal request caesareans

If there is no clinical complication that makes a c-section necessary, the current guidance from the National Institute for Health and Care Excellence (known as 'NICE') recommends that women are offered a referral to a perinatal mental health specialist for a discussion about the reasons for requesting a caesarean section. If a woman continues to request a c-section it should be performed.

Can I be refused a caesarean?

Individual obstetricians are entitled to refuse to perform a c-section in the absence of clinical need, but the guidance states that they should refer you to another obstetrician who is willing to carry out the operation. NICE guidance is not law and does not give you a legal entitlement to a particular treatment, but if a health professional declines to follow the guidance they should provide good and clear reasons for doing so.

While women have no statutory entitlement to any particular type of maternity care in the UK, the decisions of healthcare professionals about the care that they give to women must be lawful. That means decisions must be taken in accordance with the general principles of the law, and where the care is provided by the NHS, that includes the principles of public and human rights law.

The NICE guideline on elective c-sections without a clinical indication states that women ought to be offered a c-section after discussion and an offer of mental health support. NICE guidelines are not legally binding on medical professionals. However, where a decision is made to depart from a guideline, reasons need to be given and exceptions considered in each individual case.

Birth partners

Who is a birth partner?

A birth partner is a person you choose to have with you during your labour, in addition to any health professionals. Many women choose the baby's father to be their birth partner, but birth partners can also be same-sex partners, family members, friends or professional birth supporters such as doulas. You may choose not to have a birth partner, or to have more than one, and you may wish to have different birth partners at different stages of your labour.

Right to choose your birth partner

Those caring for you should respect your choice of birth partner or partners during your labour. Article 8 of the European Convention on Human Rights protects every person's right to make choices about their private life and this includes choices about birth partners.

You should be given proper opportunities to explain who you wish to be with you during your labour. Your choices should be carefully considered by midwives and other medical staff and should not be restricted or refused unless there is a good reason to do so in your individual case.

In order for a hospital's reason to be a good one, there must be a legitimate need being met by any restriction on choice of birth partner, and that restriction must be a proportionate way to meet that need. An example of a good reason might be if a birth partner has previously been violent towards health professionals.

Hospital policies

Hospitals sometimes have a policy on how many birth partners are 'permitted' in the labour room, or a policy that discourages birth partners swapping over during a woman's labour. These policies are not good reasons to limit your choices in themselves, because they do not take your individual circumstances into account. Whenever a hospital policy is applied to you, health professionals must take account of your personal needs and consider making exceptions to the policy if they are required.

Health professionals have specific obligations towards women from 'protected groups' in the Equality Act 2010. These include disabled women and women from different ethnic backgrounds. Any policy on birth partners must take particular account of the needs of women in these protected groups.

Professional birth partners

You may decide to choose a professional birth partner such as a doula or an independent midwife to provide emotional support and advocacy in labour. Doulas are birth partners who have usually received training to support women during childbirth. A doula's role is to offer physical and emotional support during labour. They are not midwives and a doula must not assume the role of a midwife. If she does so, then she could commit a criminal offence.

Independent midwives are midwives who work privately outside the NHS. In hospitals, independent midwives are not usually allowed to provide midwifery care, but they may support you and advocate on your behalf. Hospitals should respect your choice of professional birth partner in the same way that they respect your choice to have a family member or another person present during your labour.

Birth partners and consenting to medical treatment

If you have the mental capacity to make your own decisions about your health and body then you have the right to make decisions about your treatment yourself. A birth partner cannot give consent on your behalf, but they may help you make your wishes known by speaking up for you to health professionals. In an emergency, if you are unable to make your wishes known and there is time, your next-of-kin (who may also be a birth partner) should be involved in decisions about your care.

Birth partners can only consent to medical treatment for the baby if they also have parental responsibility. You can find a summary of parental responsibility on the NHS Choices website.

After your baby's birth

Hospitals sometimes have a policy about whether and for how long birth partners can stay with you after the birth of your baby. There may be good reasons for limiting birth partners on postnatal wards (such as not wanting men on women-only wards). However, those caring for you should apply the policy flexibly and sensitively to your individual circumstances.

You should be given opportunities to explain if you have particular reasons for wanting your birth partner to stay. These could include having had a c-section, or a difficult or upsetting birth, or because you need help with breastfeeding. Hospital staff should take your wishes and individual circumstances into account in deciding whether to apply the general policy, and they should make an exception unless there is a good reason not to do so. If there are ways to accommodate your request, such as providing a room off the ward, these should be considered.

Foreign nationals and maternity care
Who can receive maternity care in the UK?

Any woman in the UK can receive maternity care from the NHS regardless of her citizenship or immigration status.

Is maternity care free to all women?

Like NHS treatment generally, maternity care is free of charge to those who are 'ordinarily resident' in the UK. This can include foreign nationals. It may exclude British citizens if they do not ordinarily reside in the UK.

If you are not ordinarily resident, you may be charged for your care under the National Health Service Act 2006 and the National Health Service (Charges to Overseas Visitors) Regulations 2011. However, maternity care, even in early pregnancy, must not be withheld or delayed if a pregnant woman is unable to pay in advance, because of the health risks associated with pregnancy and childbirth. You should be informed if charges apply to your care and the NHS may pursue the debt.

What is ordinary residence?

Ordinary residence is a concept that has been developed by the courts. It is not defined in legislation. According to the courts' definition, ordinary residence requires a person to live in the UK lawfully and voluntarily and as part of the regular order of their life, with an identifiable purpose for their residence here which has a sufficient degree of continuity to be properly described as settled (R v Barnet London Borough

Council, Ex p Nilish Shah, 1983). This will include people who normally live in the UK and are not simply visiting for a temporary period.

It is up to the relevant NHS body (usually a hospital's Overseas Visitors Manager) to decide whether the criteria for ordinary residence are met in each case. Department of Health guidance provides advice on the way that ordinary residence should be established in practice, and how those who are not ordinarily resident should be identified. There is no minimum period of residence, but the Department of Health suggests that someone who has been in the UK for less than 6 months is less likely to be 'settled' than someone who has been here longer.

Are there exemptions from charging?

Yes. Under the Charging Regulations you may be exempt from charges for maternity care, even though you are not ordinarily resident in the UK. If you have been living lawfully in the UK for the past 12 months, or you are working for a UK organisation or you are self-employed in the UK, you will not be charged. A full list of categories of people who are exempted is available on NHS Choices. They include refugees, asylum seekers and victims of human trafficking. Visitors from the European Economic Area will not be charged for maternity care. Some other countries have reciprocal healthcare arrangements with the UK, which entitle their citizens to free maternity treatment. A full list of those countries is available from NHS Choices.[89]

Is treatment for any other health conditions free of charge?

Some health services are exempt from charge and free to everyone. These are:

- treatment given in an accident and emergency (A&E) department or in an NHS walk-in centre that provides services similar to those of an A&E department;
- treatment for certain infectious diseases, including HIV and AIDS.
- compulsory psychiatric treatment;
- treatment for a sexually transmitted disease; and
- family planning services.

Maternity care and pregnancy terminations are not classified as family planning services.

In order to comply with human rights obligations, treatment which is considered by doctors to be 'immediately necessary' or 'urgent' must never be withheld from overseas visitors pending payment, although charges will still apply unless the service provided is exempt from charges, as listed above. HIV treatment to prevent mother-to-child transmission of HIV is considered 'immediately necessary', and should not be withheld pending payment.

Treatment which is not covered in the list above and is not immediately necessary or urgent, will not be provided without payment in advance. Maternity care will usually be considered immediately necessary or urgent and therefore will not be withheld or delayed if a pregnant woman is unable to pay in advance.

What care can a newborn baby receive?

Care for a newborn baby will be classified as 'immediately necessary' and provided without requirement for payment in advance. If one of the baby's parents is ordinarily resident and the baby will be living with that parent, the baby will be considered ordinarily resident and the parents will not be charged for his/her care. The baby will not be ordinarily resident in the UK if neither parent is ordinarily resident and the mother will be charged for the baby's care, but it cannot be withheld pending payment.

Can pregnant visitors book with a GP?

Yes. The Department of Health guidance on charging explains that GPs have discretion to accept any person, including overseas visitors, to be either fully registered as an NHS patient, or as a temporary resident, if they are to be in an area for between 24 hours and three months.

There is no minimum period that a person needs to have been in the UK before a GP can register them. GPs have a duty to provide free of charge treatment that they consider to be immediately necessary or an emergency, regardless of whether that patient is an overseas visitor or registered with that practice.

Unassisted birth

What is unassisted birth?

Unassisted birth, often called 'freebirth', is the term used to describe a woman's decision to give birth at home or elsewhere without the assistance of a healthcare professional. It does not refer to giving birth at home before the planned arrival of a healthcare professional, known as 'born before arrival'. A woman who chooses to birth unassisted may have family members or a doula present.

Is unassisted birth legal?

Yes. Women are not obliged to accept any medical or midwifery care or treatment during childbirth and cannot be compelled to accept care unless they lack mental capacity.

Can I face sanctions for giving birth without assistance?

You cannot face any legal sanctions for giving birth without assistance. However, some healthcare professionals may believe that you are placing your unborn child at risk and that your decision raises a 'child protection' or 'safeguarding' issue, and might threaten to make a referral to social services.

Healthcare professionals should not refer a woman to social services solely on the basis that she has declined medical support, as she is legally entitled to do. Social services referrals ought to be based on an assessment of whether there is a significant risk of harm to the child after it is born. If a referral to social services is made on the basis that a pregnant woman has declined medical attention, social services will decide whether to instigate a child protection investigation.

Can my birth partner be prosecuted for supporting me?

Article 45 of the Nursing and Midwifery Order makes it a criminal offence for anyone other than a registered midwife or doctor to 'attend' a woman during childbirth, except in an emergency. This offence is not intended to prevent birth partners from supporting women, but they must ensure that they do not assume the role of a midwife by performing midwifery functions, such as monitoring the progress of labour.

The Nursing and Midwifery Council has produced guidance on this issue, which states that birth partners, including doulas and family members, 'may be present during childbirth but must not assume responsibility, assist or assume the role of the medical practitioner or registered midwife or give midwifery or medical care in childbirth.' A person convicted for this offence cannot be imprisoned, but they may incur a fine of up to £5,000.

Facing criticism: child protection, social services and maternity care

Your choices

You may find that you face criticism for the choices you make during your pregnancy and birth. Healthcare professionals or others might suggest that the choices you have made could harm your unborn child, or even that there is a 'child protection' or 'safeguarding' issue.

What is child protection in England and Wales?

Child protection describes the wide range of actions that can be taken by local authority Children's Services departments, known as social services, to intervene in families when children are believed to be at risk of 'significant harm'. It is the overall responsibility of the Department for Education, which provides guidance to social services, which are responsible for planning and providing child protection services. The Children Act 2004 established Local Safeguarding Children's Boards, which ensure that the key agencies involved in safeguarding children work effectively together.

Child protection principles are enshrined in the Children Act 1989. Government guidance 'Working Together to Safeguard Children' (2015) is the core government guidance on inter-agency cooperation to promote child protection. It is intended to provide a national framework within which local agencies and professionals agree on their own practices.

Does it apply to unborn children?

In the UK, unborn children are not given legal recognition. However, child protection procedures can apply to parents-to-be if there is a reasonable belief that the baby will be at risk of significant harm when it is born.

What does 'significant harm' mean?

The legal term 'significant harm' is defined in the Children Act 1989. It includes physical and non-physical ill-treatment and impairment of a child's health or development. The guidance explains that there are no absolute criteria for determining what constitutes significant harm. The decision about whether a child is at risk is a decision that will be made by local social services departments. If they decide to start child protection proceedings, that decision can be challenged in a court.

There is no national guidance on what constitutes a risk of harm to an unborn child. Local Safeguarding Children's Boards and social services departments have varied protocols on protecting unborn children. Common issues often identified in these protocols include:

- maternal drug and alcohol dependence
- domestic violence
- parent aged under 16
- parent who has previously harmed a child
- previous unexplained death of a child where abuse or neglect is suspected
- denial of pregnancy
- avoidance of antenatal care, and
- non-cooperation with healthcare services and/or non-compliance with medical treatment.

How are child protection concerns reported?

Anyone, including members of the public, can refer concerns about the welfare of a child to their local authority child protection team. Healthcare organisations have designated individuals who deal with child protection issues, and procedures for referring concerns to social services. They will have clear policies on how such issues should be dealt with and when they should be referred. Healthcare professionals, including doctors, midwives and health visitors, are expected by their professional bodies to know what to do if they have concerns about risk to an unborn child and to act in accordance with national and local child protection policies.

Child protection policies require healthcare professionals to discuss concerns with parents-to-be and obtain their consent before a referral to children's services, unless this action in itself may place the welfare of the unborn child at risk.

Can a referral be based on my birth choices?

Child protection policies sometimes suggest that healthcare professionals should make a referral to social services when they consider that a woman's choices about medical care during her birth put her unborn child at risk. Referral to social services would be inappropriate unless the mother's choices indicated that there was a threat of significant harm to the baby once it was born.

If you have made an informed decision to refuse care or to birth outside hospital, you cannot be compelled to accept care unless you lack mental capacity to make your own decisions about medical treatment. The threat of referral to social services should never be used to intimidate, bully or coerce you into accepting a particular medical intervention for you or your child.

Consent given on the basis of such a threat is not given freely, and the healthcare professional may be legally liable for battery and violation of Article 8 of the European Convention if they perform the intervention and they know, or should know, that consent has not been freely given.

What happens if child protection concerns are reported?

After a referral is made to a local authority the guidance

states that an initial assessment must be carried out within 10 working days in accordance with the Local Safeguarding Children's Board's procedures. These procedures vary across the country, but they should always be publicly available for any person who wishes to access them. If, following the initial assessment, the baby is judged to be at risk of significant harm, professionals from relevant agencies will meet to decide whether to initiate an enquiry under section 47 of the Children Act 1989.

Section 47 enquiries

Section 47 enquiries are based on a 'core assessment'. This involves gathering more information from the parents, family members and other professionals in order to determine whether the baby is at risk of significant harm. The core assessment is the responsibility of the social worker, but information from other agencies, such as hospitals, will be collected and analysed. Parents must be consulted in a section 47 enquiry, unless their involvement would increase the risk to the unborn child. If parents refuse to cooperate or provide information, a local authority can apply to the court for a child assessment order. In these circumstances, the court may direct the parents to cooperate with an assessment.

Child protection conferences

If the section 47 assessment concludes that the baby is at risk of significant harm, an initial, pre-birth, child protection conference will be arranged. The conference brings together family members and professionals involved with the family. Its purpose is to analyse the information which has been obtained; to make judgements about the likelihood of the baby suffering significant harm in the future; and to decide what future action is required in order to safeguard and promote the welfare of the baby. The guidance gives advice on holding pre-birth child protection conferences. It states that the involvement of midwifery services is 'vital'. The conference must proceed in the same way as any other child protection conference, including deciding during the conference whether to make a 'child protection plan'.

Child protection plans

A child protection plan should be made in the conference if there is reason to suspect that the unborn baby may be at continuing risk of significant harm. The plan must consider the immediate safety needs of the child once it is born, as well as future needs and details of any further assessments required. The plan must explain what action social services intend to take after the birth of the child, including whether they intend to seek an emergency protection order from the court removing the child from its parents at birth.

If a child protection plan is made, the child's name will be placed on the Child Protection Register. A further child protection conference will be held after the child is born to decide whether any action needs to be taken to protect the child.

Care proceedings

'Care proceedings' is the phrase used to describe the legal process by which social services ask the court whether or not a child should be taken into care. If a court decides that a child should go into care this is called making a 'care order'.

Care proceedings cannot be started before a baby is born. In rare circumstances, and particularly where there has not been time to prepare an application for an interim care order (see below), if it is felt that a baby will be in immediate danger at birth, social services can apply to the court for an 'emergency protection order' as soon as the baby is born. If an emergency protection order is granted, the baby can be removed from its parents shortly after birth for up to eight days. The order may be extended if needed.

If social services intend to take the baby into care for the long term, they will ask the court to make 'interim care orders' while matters are investigated further and plans made. Interim care orders are made for eight weeks at first, and must be renewed every four weeks. If, after investigation, social services still think a care order is necessary, they will ask the court to make a full care order.

A court will only make a care order if it finds that the child is suffering, or is likely to suffer, significant harm, and that the harm is attributable to the parents or carers. The court may decide that a less interventionist order is appropriate, for example providing for supervision of the child by social services, or restricting the exercise of parental responsibility while leaving the child in the care of its parents. The court must be convinced that making an order is better for the child than making no order at all.

Can I make a complaint?

If you feel that a healthcare professional has acted inappropriately by threatening you or making a referral to social services, you can make a complaint to that individual's employer. NHS organisations will have people responsible for dealing with complaints. If you are unhappy with the outcome of a complaint, you can refer the matter to the Parliamentary and Health Service Ombudsman.

If your complaint is about a social worker you can complain to the local authority social services department. They will have a formal complaints procedure. If you wish to complain about a child protection conference then you should make a complaint to the chair of the conference or their manager. If you are still unhappy you can make a complaint to the Local Government Ombudsman.

Complaints should be made as soon as possible after the event being complained about. The NHS and social services departments ask for complaints to be made within 12 months unless there is a good reason why you could not have complained sooner. You can find more information about challenging decisions and making a complaint on the Family Rights Group website.

Accessing your records

What are my maternity records?

If you receive NHS maternity care in the UK you will receive a set of maternity records, often called your handheld records, at your booking appointment, which you keep with you throughout your pregnancy and birth. In future these may become electronic records which you and your caregivers can access from a range of places and devices.

Midwives and doctors make a note of all the maternity care they provide in the records, including test and scan results. After your baby's birth and discharge from hospital, these records are retained by the hospital. Some hospitals now use electronic systems for making notes during labour. Some hospitals may print out these records and add them to the blue book, but practice varies across hospitals.

If you have given birth at home under NHS care, the records will be taken by the midwife who has attended you and she will give them to the local hospital. If you have used private maternity care – either an independent midwife or a private obstetrician – your care provider will retain a copy of your notes. Healthcare records are also made about your baby, once they are born.

How can I obtain my records?

You can ask your GP, midwife, doctor or health visitor informally, at any time, whether they can obtain your records for you to view in person at the GP's surgery or hospital. You have a right under the Data Protection Act 1998 to access your own health records. You can submit a formal written request, known as a 'subject access request', to view your notes under the Data Protection Act 1998. This is usually sent to the NHS Trust's medical records manager or the GP surgery's practice manager. The address will be available on the relevant NHS Trust or surgery website. You and your partner, if they have parental responsibility for your child, have a right of access to your child's medical records. The Information Commissioner provides standard letters that you can use to make a request.

How long will it take?

Subject access requests must be processed within 40 days. The NHS is committed to providing healthcare records within 21 days. If you are considering making a complaint, it may be helpful to write down your own recollection of events while you wait to receive your records.

Can I be refused access to my records?

Access can be refused on two grounds: if the person holding the records believes that providing the information may cause serious harm to the patient's physical or mental health; or if access would disclose information relating to a third party (non-healthcare professional), unless the third party consents or it is reasonable to disclose the information.

It is very unlikely that either of these grounds would apply to maternity records. If you encounter any difficulties obtaining your notes, you can make a complaint to the Information Commissioner's Office.

Is there a fee?

A fee (not more than £50) is usually payable if you require copies of your notes and a fee (not more than £10) may also be charged for viewing the notes. If the notes have been added to in the last 40 days, viewing should be free. Details of the fees are available on the NHS Choices website. The fee is discretionary and intended to cover administrative costs, such as photocopying. You have a right to access to medical information that is held about you under Article 8 of the European Convention on Human Rights, so if you cannot afford to pay for your records and you can show that you are on a low income, the hospital ought to waive the fee.

Can I photograph my records before I am discharged?

Women are sometimes informed that they are not allowed to photograph their notes before they leave the hospital and that they must make a formal request under the Data Protection Act. Your maternity records are officially owned by the NHS Trust and they are entitled to control whether copies are made. You can ask at any time during your care to view your records informally without making a subject access request.

Can I amend my records?

The Data Protection Act requires that all records are factually accurate and up to date. If you discover an inaccuracy in your records, you can request an appointment with the health professional who made the record and ask for it to be amended. If they do not accept that the record is inaccurate, you should be permitted to include a written statement in the record stating that you disagree with it.

How long are records retained?

Your maternity records and your child's records must be retained for 25 years after the birth of your child.

How can I interpret my records?

Once you have the records, you may want to go through them with a health professional in order to understand any jargon or technical references. If you are not comfortable approaching your GP, health visitor, midwife or consultant, you can ask an independent midwife to go through them with you, but you may be charged a fee. You can find details of local independent midwives through Independent Midwives UK.

Making a complaint
Your right to make a complaint

The NHS Constitution guarantees every patient the right to make a complaint about NHS services, and the NHS is bound by a statutory complaints procedure. All complaints must be dealt with efficiently and must be properly investigated. You have a right to know the outcome of any investigation and to take your complaint to the independent Health Service Ombudsman if you are not satisfied with the way your complaint has been dealt with by the NHS.

Raising concerns before you give birth

If you have concerns about your maternity care before you give birth, such as access to out-of-hospital care, entitlement to pain relief or postnatal arrangements, you should raise these as soon as you can with your healthcare professional and their manager. If you need further assistance, you can contact a Supervisor of Midwives or the Local Supervisory Authority Midwifery Officer.

Birthrights offers a free and confidential legal advice service for women and healthcare professionals seeking advice about provision of maternity care of all varieties. You can contact them by email: info@birthrights.org.uk.

Birth afterthoughts

In some areas, NHS midwives run a 'birth afterthoughts' service, which offers an opportunity to go through your notes and experience and try to resolve any unanswered questions you may have about them. These services also give hospital trusts a chance to resolve queries, which may otherwise escalate into complaints. Your local Patient Advice and Liaison Service (PALS) should be able to tell you whether a birth afterthoughts scheme operates in your area.

Before you make a complaint

If you are considering making a complaint, you may want to make a note of your experience as soon as you can. You could also ask anyone who was present with you to write down what they witnessed and give you a copy.

Before you make a complaint, it is always a good idea to request a copy of your and/or your baby's healthcare records. You should generally wait to receive the records before you make a complaint, as you may have a better understanding of what happened and who was involved in your care once you have seen your notes.

Who do I complain to?

If you have a complaint about maternity care you received from the NHS, you can complain to the NHS body responsible for your care. This will generally be a hospital trust, your GP, or an ambulance trust. NHS trusts provide details of who to contact locally on their websites.

You may also wish to complain to a professional body such as the General Medical Council, where the complaint relates to a doctor, or the Nursing and Midwifery Council where it relates to a midwife or nurse. You could consider complaining to the NHS body that commissioned the maternity care you received, particularly if your complaint relates to policies or provision of a service or treatment, rather than the conduct of an individual health professional. Clinical Commissioning Groups are responsible for commissioning care in England.

Writing your complaint

You should address your complaint to the chief executive of the NHS trust, or the GP practice manager. You may also want to copy your complaint to the head of midwifery, director of women's services, director of nursing, chief executive and/ or the consultant responsible for your care (if any). Your complaint should be as detailed as possible and provide the names of the people involved in your care, if you know them. It is useful to use numbered points in your complaint so that you can make sure that the care provider has addressed all the issues you have raised.

The complaints process

The NHS statutory complaints procedure sets out the process that must be followed when dealing with a complaint. NHS trusts also produce their own local procedures, which are based on the statutory procedure. Your local Patient Advice and Liaison Service (PALS) should be able to provide a copy of the NHS trust's complaints procedure and contact details.

Once you have made a complaint, you should receive an acknowledgement from the care provider within 2–3 working days, confirming that your complaint has been received and indicating what will happen next.

NHS bodies are obliged to investigate your complaint speedily and efficiently and keep you informed as to the progress of the investigation. You may be invited to a meeting at the hospital, surgery or clinic to discuss your complaint.

You can ask for the meeting to be held at your own home or a neutral venue if that would make you more comfortable. It is a good idea to take someone who was not involved in your birth with you to the meeting.

The response to your complaint must usually be sent within six months of the complaint being made. You should receive an explanation of how the complaint has been considered and the conclusions reached, including whether the care provider intends to take any remedial action, such as disciplinary action against staff or changes to its policies or practice.

If the care provider accepts that mistakes were made in your care, they should apologise. You cannot be offered compensation through the complaints process.

Is there a time limit for making a complaint?

A formal complaint under the NHS complaints procedure must be made within 12 months of the date of treatment. If you discover a reason for making a complaint after the 12 months have elapsed, you can make a complaint within 12 months of that date. The deadline may be extended where the person making the complaint had good reasons for not doing so within the time limit and it is still possible to investigate the complaint fairly and effectively. In the context of maternity services, it may well be the case that birth trauma prevents you from making your complaint within a year, and you should not be put off from making a complaint outside the time limit.

You could consider writing to the care provider before the 12 months elapses to inform them that you intend to make a complaint when you are well enough to do so.

The Health Service Ombudsman

If the relevant NHS body has not satisfactorily resolved your complaint, you can refer it to the Parliamentary and Health

Service Ombudsman in England or the Public Services Ombudsman in Wales.

The Ombudsman will usually only accept a complaint if attempts to resolve it at a local level with the relevant NHS body have been unsuccessful and it does not have to investigate your complaint. Complaints should be referred to the Ombudsman as soon as possible and within a year of the incident. The Ombudsman can extend this deadline if attempts at resolution have delayed submission of the complaint. If you are unhappy with the way that the NHS body handled your complaint, you can include this in your complaint to the Ombudsman.

Complaints to professional bodies

You can also complain about an individual member of staff to their professional body on the grounds that they are not fit to practise. Complaints about midwives and/or nurses can be made to the Nursing and Midwifery Council, and complaints about doctors to the General Medical Council.

You can also raise concerns about a midwife with the Supervisor of Midwives or the Local Supervisory Authority Midwifery Officer. Professional bodies usually expect the employer (i.e. the NHS body) to try to resolve the issue before they get involved in any complaint.

Taking legal action

You may be able to take legal action in relation to negligent treatment or any breach of your rights, subject to the limitation periods set out below. The court will expect you to have exhausted other avenues to resolve your complaint (such as the NHS complaint process and referral to the Ombudsman) before starting legal action.

Any claim by or on behalf of the mother must be issued

within three years of the birth. The child will usually be able to claim until their 21st birthday. Legal action is often expensive and you may not recover all of your costs. It is advisable to seek independent legal advice before launching a claim. Many solicitors' firms offer a free initial assessment of personal injury claims. Action against Medical Accidents is a charity that promotes better patient safety and justice for people who have suffered avoidable harm. It offers free and confidential advice and support, including a helpline. The Citizens Advice Bureau also offers guidance on taking legal action and making a complaint about care. The NHS Litigation Authority also provides some information on how negligence claims are handled.

> This guide was taken from the Birthrights Factsheets
> available at www.birthrights.org.uk

Your rights outside the UK
International
Human Rights in Childbirth:
www.humanrightsinchildbirth.org
Human Rights in Childbirth provides information on the six universal rights that impact on childbearing women across the world. Their regional networks can provide support and information in your area. They are developing 'know your rights' factsheets for a number of countries without such resources.

White Ribbon Alliance: whiteribbonalliance.org/wp-content/uploads/2013/10/Final_RMC_Charter.pdf
The WRA's Charter on the universal rights of childbearing women is useful in all countries for pregnant women and those who care for them.

USA
Childbirth Connections: www.childbirthconnection.org
'The Rights of Childbearing Women' sets out women's basic
rights in pregnancy, birth and the postnatal period in the US.

National Advocates for Pregnant Women:
www.advocatesforpregnantwomen.org
NAPW seeks to protect the rights and human dignity of
all women, particularly pregnant and parenting women
and those who are most vulnerable including low-income
women, women of colour, and drug-using women. They may
be able to provide legal assistance.

Improving Birth: improvingbirth.org
Improving Birth advocate for respectful, evidence-based care
in the US. They are working on a summary of women's civil
rights in childbirth at the moment and have an emergency
contact form for women whose rights are being violated in
childbirth or who are being threatened by the courts, police
or Child Protective Services for a pregnancy or birth-related
reason.

South America
The Stork Network:
dab.saude.gov.br/portaldab/ape_redecegonha.
php?conteudo=caderneta_gestante
The Network has a range of information (in Portuguese)
for health care professionals and a handbook for pregnant
women.

Australia
Maternity Choice Australia:
www.maternitychoices.org.au
Maternity Choices Australia, formally Maternity Coalition
(MC) is a national consumer advocacy organisation
committed to the advancement of best-practice maternity care
for all Australian women and their families.

New Zealand
Birthmatters:
birthmatters.co.nz/category/issues-of-birth-rights

Hungary
Tasz: Fundamental Rights of Birthing Women: tasz.hu/
betegjog/szulo-nok-alapveto-jogai

Slovakia
Women's Human Rights in Obstetric Care in Healthcare
Facilities in Slovakia:
odz.sk/en/women-mothers-bodies

Croatia
Prirodan Porod: www.prirodanporod.com

Portugal
Portuguese Association for Women's Rights in Pregnancy
and Childbirth www.associacaogravidezeparto.pt/
sombrasdoparto.wordpress.com

Further Reading and Resources

Further reading on human rights

Clapham, Andrew. *Human Rights*. Oxford: Oxford University Press, 2007

Chakrabarti, Shami. *On Liberty*. London: Penguin, 2015

We Are All Born Free. London: Frances Lincoln Children's Books in association with Amnesty International, 2008

Hunt, Lynn. *Inventing Human Rights*. W.W. Norton & Company, 2008

Further reading on women's rights and feminism

Feminist Doulas and Midwives and Obstetricians Facebook Group: www.facebook.com/groups/576122959129565

Worden, Minky. *An Unfinished Revolution*. Policy Press, 2012

Joachim, Jutta M. *Agenda Setting, The UN, And NGOs*. Washington, D.C.: Georgetown University Press, 2007

Feldt, Gloria, and Laura Fraser. *The War On Choice*. New York: Bantam Books, 2004

Further reading on childbirth and rights

Beech, Beverley A. Lawrence. *Am I Allowed?* Surbiton, Surrey, England: Association for Improvements in the Maternity Services, 2014. Print

References: Further Reading and Resources

Support for women in the UK

Birthrights: www.birthrights.org.uk

Association for the Improvement of Maternity Services: AIMS.org.uk

Maternity Action: www.maternityaction.org.uk

Pregnant Then Screwed: pregnantthenscrewed.com

Patient Advice and Liaison Service: www.patients-association.org.uk/helpline

Positive Birth Movement: www.positivebirthmovement.org

Birth Trauma Association: www.birthtraumaassociation.org.uk

London Trauma Specialists (specialists in birth trauma recovery): londontraumaspecialists.com

British Pregnancy Advisory Service: www.bpas.org

Planned Caesarean Section Support Group: www.facebook.com/groups/178142412343271

Independent Midwives UK: imuk.org.uk

Doula UK: doula.org.uk

The Independent Complaints Advocacy Service: nhscomplaintsadvocacy.org

There are a number of Facebook support groups for unassisted birth. To protect their members these are not listed here.

International support for women

Midwives for Choice (Ireland): midwivesforchoice.ie

Human Rights in Childbirth (Global): www.humanrightsinchildbirth.org

Childbirth Connections (USA): www.childbirthconnection.org

National Advocates for Pregnant Women (USA): www.advocatesforpregnantwomen.org

Improving Birth (USA): improvingbirth.org

The Stork Network (Brazil): dab.saude.gov.br/portaldab/ape_redecegonha.php?conteudo=caderneta_gestante

Maternity Choice Australia: www.maternitychoices.org.au

Tasz (Hungary): Fundamental Rights of Birthing Women tasz.hu/betegjog/szulo-nok-alapveto-jogai

El Parto Es Nuestro (Spain): www.elpartoesnuestro.es

There are a number of Facebook support groups for unassisted birth. To protect their members these are not listed here.

Resources and information for healthcare professionals

- Birthrights will be producing a series of short videos on respectful maternity care in 2016. These will be available at birthrights.org.uk
- Also forthcoming in 2016 is a Royal College of Midwives/ Birthrights online self-study module. This will be available to RCM members at www.ilearn.rcm.org.uk
- For details of Birthrights' free and bespoke training for midwives and doctors see: birthrights.org.uk
- Disrespect and Abuse during Childbirth: Emerging Evidence to Inform Policy Advocacy, a webinar by CHANGE, available at vimeo.com/111680764
- The International MotherBaby Childbirth Organization: 10 Steps to Optimal Maternity Services: www.imbci.org
- Obstetric Violence in Mexico: www.youtube.com/ watch?v=kZgLJ_MYQmo
- Obstetric Violence and Human Rights, a lecture by Consultant Obstetrician Amali Lokugamage: www.youtube. com/watch?v=Ziy5kSFm7U8
- White Ribbon Alliance's Charter on Respectful Maternity Care: whiteribbonalliance.org/wp-content/uploads/2013/10/ Final_RMC_Charter.pdf
- New Zealand College of Midwives: www.midwife.org.nz
- Royal College of Midwives Better Births Campaign: www. rcm.org.uk/better-births-initiative
- Elizabeth Prochaska addresses the launch of Midwives for Choice: www.youtube.com/watch?v=bOVDK7zcVkM

References

Chapter 1

1. Save the Children, 'Missing Midwives' (2011), p.vii

Chapter 2

2. McIntosh, T., *A Social History of Maternity and Childbirth* (London: Routledge, 2012)
3. 'Our "mommy" problem', available at: mobile.nytimes.com/2014/11/09/ opinion/sunday/our-mommy-problem.html?referrer&_r=3 [accessed 15 January 2016]
4. L'Estrange, E., 'En/Gendering representations of childbirth in fifteenth-century franco-flemish devotional manuscripts' (PhD Thesis, 2003)
5. Brennecke, S. et al., 'Diminished hERG K+ channel activity facilitates strong human labour contractions but is dysregulated in obese women', *Nature Communications* (2014), Article 4108, Vol. 5
6. Mendelson, C., 'Minireview: fetal-maternal hormonal signaling in pregnancy and labor', *Molecular Endocrinology* (2009), 23(7), pp. 947–54
7. 'Long-held theory on human gestation refuted: Mother's metabolism, not birth canal size, limits gestation', available at: www.sciencedaily.com/ releases/2012/08/120827152037.htm [accessed 21 March 2016]
8. Uvnäs Moberg, K., *The Oxytocin Factor* (London: Pinter & Martin Ltd, 2011)
9. Odent, M., *Childbirth in the Age of Plastics* (London: Pinter & Martin Ltd, 2011)
10. One World Birth, *MicroBirth* (2014): www.oneworldbirth.net/microbirth
11. Albert, E., 'Confessions of a radical doula', available at: nymag.com/ thecut/2016/03/confessions-of-a-radical-doula-c-v-r.html [accessed 5 July 2016]
12. Green, J. *et al.*, 'Greater Expectations?' (2003): www.york.ac.uk/media/ healthsciences/documents/miru/GreaterExpdf.pdf
13. Kitzinger, S., *Freedom and Choice in Childbirth* (Harmondsworth: Penguin, 1988)
14. Better Births: Improving Outcome of Maternity Services in England, available at www.england.nhs.uk/wp-content/uploads/2016/02/ national-maternity-review-report.pdf [accessed on 17 March 2016]
15. 'Midwives, not medicine, rule pregnancy in Sweden', available at: www.

nydailynews.com/life-style/health/midwives-medicine-rule-pregnancy-sweden-article-1.1478407 [accessed 21 March 2016]

16. De Jonge, A., Mesman, J., Manniën, J., Zwart, J., Van Dillen, J. and Van Roosmalen, J., 'Severe adverse maternal outcomes among low risk women with planned home versus hospital births in the Netherlands: nationwide cohort study', *BMJ* (2013), 346: f3263

17. Australian Homebirth Statistics, available at: homebirthaustralia.org/statistics [accessed 20 February 2016]

18. Data available at: www.hscic.gov.uk/pubs/maternity1011 [accessed 21 March 2016]

19. Lauria, L., Lamberti, A., Buoncristiano, M., Bonciani, M. and Andreozzi, S., 'Percorso nascita: promozione e valutazione della qualità di modelli operativi. Le indagini del 2008-2009 e del 2010-2011', Rapporti ISTISAN, No. 12/39 (Roma: Istituto Superiore di Sanità – Centro Nazionale di Epidemiologia, 2012). Retrieved from: www.iss.it/binary/publ/cont/12_39_web.pdf

20. EURO-PERISTAT project with SCPE and EUROCAT: European Perinatal Health Report, 'The health and care of pregnant women and babies in Europe in 2010' (May 2013), available at: www.europeristat.com

21. Data available at indicators.rcog.org.uk

22. Hollowell, J., 'Birthplace programme overview: background, component studies and summary of findings' – Birthplace in England research programme. Final report part 1 (2011, updated 2014). NIHR Service Delivery and Organisation programme

23. Edited from Meaghan O'Connell, Longreads Blog, available at: blog.longreads.com/tag/meaghan-oconnell [accessed 26 November 2014]

24. Simkin, P., 'Just another day in a woman's life? Part II: Nature and consistency of women's long-term memories of their first birth experiences', *Birth* (1992), 19(2), pp. 64–81

25. Takehara, K., Noguchi, M., Shimane, T. and Misago, C., 'A longitudinal study of women's memories of their childbirth experiences at five years postpartum', *BMC Pregnancy and Childbirth* (2014), 14(1), p. 221

26. Dignity Survey, available at: www.birthrights.org.uk/campaigns/dignity-in-childbirth/dignity-survey [accessed 6 July 2016]

27. 'Saving mothers' lives: reviewing maternal deaths to make motherhood safer: 2006–2008', *BJOG: An International Journal of Obstetrics & Gynaecology* (2011), Vol. 118, pp. 1–203

Chapter 3

28. Clapham, Andrew. *Human Rights.* Oxford: Oxford University Press, 2007

29. www.justice.gov.uk/downloads/human-rights/human-rights-making-sense-human-rights.pdf (Accessed March 2016)

30. United Nations Convention on the Elimination of All Forms,of Discrimination against Women (47th session, 2010), 'Concluding observations of the Committee on the Elimination of Discrimination against Women', available at www2.ohchr.org/english/bodies/cedaw/docs/co/CEDAW-C-CZE-CO-5.pdf [accessed 26 January 2015]

31. 'Perinatal and maternal outcomes by planned place of birth for healthy women with low risk pregnancies: the Birthplace in England national prospective cohort study', *BMJ* (2011), 343: d7400

32. 'The case of Dr Ágnes Geréb', Human Rights in Childbirth (2013), available at: humanrightsinchildbirth.com/the-case-of-dr-agnes-gereb/ [accessed July 2016]

33. 'National training survey 2014', General Medical Council, available at: www.gmc-uk.org/NTS_bullying_and_undermining_report_2014_FINAL.pdf_58648010.pdf [accessed July 2016]

34. Shabazz, T., Parry-Smith, W., Oates, S., *et al* Consultants as victims of bullying and undermining: a survey of Royal College of Obstetricians and Gynaecologists consultant experiences, *BMJ Open* 2016; 6: e011462. doi: 10.1136/bmjopen-2016-011462

35. NHS Staff Survey 2013, available at: www.nhsstaffsurveys.com/Page/1006/Latest-Results/2015-Results [accessed 10 July 2016]

Chapter 4

36. Kant, I., *Grounding for the Metaphysics of Morals* (New York: BN Publishing, 2010)

37. 'Prevention and elimination of disrespect and abuse during childbirth', WHO (2014), available at: www.who.int/reproductivehealth/topics/maternal_perinatal/statement-childbirth/en [accessed July 2016]

38. D'Oliveira, A., Diniz, S. and Schraiber, L., 'Violence against women in health-care institutions: an emerging problem', *The Lancet* (2002), 359(9318), pp. 1681–5.

39. Names have been changed to protect the individuals involved

40. 'National Maternity Services Plan', Australian Government Department of Health (2010), available at: www.health.gov.au/internet/main/publishing.nsf/Content/maternityservicesplan [accessed July 2016]

41. Ireland, S., Wulili Narjic, C., Belton, S. and Kildea, S., 'Niyith Nniyith

Watmam [The Quiet Story]: Exploring the experiences of Aboriginal women who give birth in their remote community', *Midwifery* (2011), 27(5), pp. 634–41

42. 'Tassie Heritage claim ignored', reader's letter, *Koori Mail*, 490, p. 24

43. 'Tell your story', *Koori Mail*, 400, p. 21

44. Van Wagner, V. et al., 'Midwifery in remote Nunavik, Quebec', Ryerson University (2012), available at: fcsktp.ryerson.ca/xmlui/handle/123456789/46 [accessed 6 December 2014]

45. 'Perinatal and maternal outcomes by planned place of birth for healthy women with low risk pregnancies: the Birthplace in England national prospective cohort study', *BMJ* (2011), 343: d7400

46. 'Home Births', RANZCOG (2014), available at: www.ranzcog.edu.au/documents/doc_view/2051-home-births-c-obs-2.html [accessed July 2016]

47. Kruske, S., Young, K., Jenkinson, B. and Catchlove, A., 'Maternity care providers' perceptions of women's autonomy and the law', *BMC Pregnancy and Childbirth* (2013), 13(1), p. 84

48. Birthrights and bpas (2014), available at: www.birthrights.org.uk/wordpress/wp-content/uploads/2014/11/BPAS-Birthrights-CP-v-CICA-Intervention.pdf [accessed 6 December 2014]

49. Laura Pemberton, Vimeo (2009), available at: vimeo.com/4895023 [accessed 7 December 2014]

Chapter 5

50. Name has been changed

51. 'A high price to pay: detention of poor patients in burundian hospitals', Human Rights Watch (2006)

52. Schutte, J., Steegers, E., Schuitemaker, N., Santema, J., De Boer, K., Pel, M., Vermeulen, G., Visser, W. and Van Roosmalen, J., 'Rise in maternal mortality in the Netherlands', *BJOG: An International Journal of Obstetrics & Gynaecology* (2010), Vol. 117(4), pp. 399–406

53. 'Saving Lives, Improving Mothers' Care', MBRRACE-UK (2014), available at: on www.npeu.ox.ac.uk/mbrrace-uk/reportsMB [accessed 26 January 2015]

54. Ebtehaj, F. *et al.* (eds.), *Birth Rites and Rights* (Oxford: Hart Publishing, 2011)

55. Wiseman, O., 'Undocumented migrants and maternity care', *Br J Midwifery* (2011), 19(1), pp. 38–42

56. Experiences of Pregnant Migrant Women receiving Ante/Peri and

Postnatal Care in the UK, Doctors of the World (2015), available at b.3cdn.net/droftheworld/5a507ef4b2316bbb07_5nm6bkfx7.pdf [accessed 16 March 2016]

57. *Br J Midwifery* (2013), available at: www.refugeecouncil.org.uk/assets/0002/8418/BJM_21_6_404-409_refugees.pdf [accessed 1 August 2016]

58. Kimberley initially went under the pseudonym of 'Kelly' to protect her identity. Thanks to: humanrightsinchildbirth.com and www.improvingbirth.org

59. Such violence is defined as: 'The appropriation of the body and reproductive processes of women by health personnel, which is expressed as dehumanised treatment, an abuse of medication, and to convert the natural processes into pathological ones, bringing with it loss of autonomy and the ability to decide freely about their bodies and sexuality, negatively impacting the quality of life of women.' It's important to add that any maternity worker or system can perpetrate this violence, not just obstetricians.

60. 'Doctor performs episiotomy despite woman's refusal', *OBG Management* (2003), available at: www.obgmanagement.com/the-latest/past-issues-single-view/doctor-performs-episiotomy-despite-womans-refusal/840a5657254d15106978d2930cbfd12a.html [accessed 3 March 2016]

61. 'Woman charges OB with assault and battery', Improving Birth (2015), available at: improvingbirth.org/2015/06/preview-woman-charges-ob-with-assault-battery-for-forced-episiotomy [accessed 10 February 2016]

62. Albert, E., 'Confessions of a radical doula', available at: nymag.com/thecut/2016/03/confessions-of-a-radical-doula-c-v-r.html [accessed 5 July 2016]

63. The full judgement is available at www.supremecourt.uk/decided-cases/docs/UKSC_2013_0136_Judgment.pdf [accessed on 21 March 2016]

64. Dignity Survey, available at: www.birthrights.org.uk/campaigns/dignity-in-childbirth/dignity-survey/ [accessed 1 August 2016]

65. Green, J. *et al.*, 'Greater Expectations?' (2003): www.york.ac.uk/media/healthsciences/documents/miru/GreaterExpdf.pdf

66. Available at www.thetimes.co.uk/tto/health/news/article4697043.ece [accessed 16 March 2016]

67. Available at www.dailymail.co.uk/health/article-3485780/Why-NO-woman-home-birth-Government-drive-free-hospital-beds-lead-rise-dead-damaged-babies-doctor-warns.html [accessed 16 March 2016]

68. Available at www.dailymail.co.uk/health/article-3493688/A-second-

Caesarean-WON-T-harm-baby.html [accessed 16 March 2016]
69. Maternity Matters, Department of Health (2007). Available at webarchive. nationalarchives.gov.uk/20130107105354/http:/www.dh.gov.uk/prod_ consum_dh/groups/dh_digitalassets/@dh/@en/documents/digitalasset/ dh_074199.pdf [accessed 16 March 2016]

Chapter 6

70. YouGov Survey (2011), available at: cdn.yougov.com/today_uk_import/ yg-archives-yougov-abortions-060911.pdf [accessed 18 February 2016]
71. Gallup Survey (2015), available at: www.gallup.com/poll/1576/abortion. aspx [accessed 23 March 2016]
72. Beech, B., 'Challenging the medicalisation of birth', *AIMS Journal* (2011), Vol. 23, No. 2
73. Ulrich, L., *A Midwife's Tale* (New York: Knopf, 1990)
74. 'Your home birth is not a feminist statement', Isis the Scientist (2011), available at: isisthescientist.com/2011/08/23/your-home-birth-is-not-a-feminist-statement [accessed July 2016]
75. Robertson, A., 'The pain of labour – a feminist issue', Birth International, available at: www.birthinternational.com/articles/midwifery/48-the-pain-of-labour-a-feminist-issue [accessed July 2016]
76. Goer, H., 'Cruelty in Maternity Wards: Fifty Years Later', *Journal of Perinatal Education* (2010), 19(3), pp. 33–42
77. Cadernos de Saúde Pública, Vol. 30, Supplement 1 (2014), available at: www.scielo.br/scielo.php?script=sci_issuetoc&pid=0102-311X20140013&lng=en&nrm=iso [accessed 8 March 2016]
78. Domingues, R., Dias, M., Nakamura-Pereira, M., Torres, J., D'Orsi, E., Pereira, A., Schilithz, A. and Leal, M., 'Processo de decisão pelo tipo de parto no Brasil: da preferência inicial das mulheres à via de parto final', Cadernos de Saúde Pública (2014), 30, S101–16
79. 'Continuous support for women during childbirth' Cochrane Summaries (2013), available at: summaries.cochrane.org/CD003766/PREG_continuous-support-for-women-during-childbirth [accessed July 2016]
80. Paltrow, L. and Flavin, J., 'Arrests of and forced interventions on pregnant women in the United States, 1973–2005: implications for women's legal status and public health', *Journal of Health Politics, Policy and Law* (2013), 38(2), pp. 299–343
81. Paltrow, L. and Flavin, J., 'Pregnant, and no civil rights', *New York Times* (2014), available at: www.nytimes.com/2014/11/08/opinion/pregnant-and-no-civil-rights.html [accessed July 2016]

82. 'Fetal homicide laws', National Conference of State Legislatures (2013), available at: www.ncsl.org/research/health/fetal-homicide-state-laws.aspx [accessed 20 February 2016]

83. 'Hearing today in foetal alcohol syndrome case', Birthrights (2014), available at: www.birthrights.org.uk/2014/11/hearing-today-in-foetal-alcohol-syndrome-case/ [accessed 16 March 2016]

84. Martin, N., 'This Alabama judge has figured out how to dismantle Roe v. Wade', ProPublica (2014), available at: www.propublica.org/article/this-alabama-judge-has-figured-out-how-to-dismantle-roe-v-wade [accessed 2 March 2016]

85. National Consent Policy, Health Service Executive (2014), available at: www.hse.ie/eng/about/Who/qualityandpatientsafety/National_Consent_Policy/consenttrainerresource/trainerfiles/NationalConsentPolicyM2014.pdf [accessed 16 March 2016]

Conclusion

86. 'Respectful maternity care: the universal rights of childbearing women', White Ribbon Alliance (2013), available at: whiteribbonalliance.org/wp-content/uploads/2013/10/Final_RMC_Charter.pdf [accessed 20 February 2016]

87. 'Intrapartum care: care of healthy women and their babies during childbirth', NICE guidelines [CG190] (2014), available at: www.nice.org.uk/guidance/CG190 [accessed 20 February 2016]

88. Stork Network – towards a new model of care, Parto Pelo Mundo (2012), available at partopelomundo.com/blog/2012/10/02/stork-network-towards-a-new-model-of-care/#sthash.3vbRKMAg.dpuf [accessed on 21 March 2016]

Further Reading and Resources

89. www.nhs.uk/NHSEngland/Healthcareabroad/countryguide/NonEEAcountries/Pages/Non-EEAcountries.aspx (accessed March 2016)

Index